WAR WITH MYSELF

ACHIEVING VICTORY IN THE BATTLE WITH BULIMIA

SHANI-LEE WALLIS

Cover Artist
TRISHA FUENTES

VALIANCE PUBLICATIONS, LLC

Printed in the United States of America
First printing: 2022
Valiance Publications, LLC
PO Box #1071
Queen Creek
AZ, 85142

DISCLAIMER

This book is designed to provide information on eating disorders and bulimia only. This information is provided and sold with the knowledge that the publisher and author do not offer any legal or other professional advice. In the case of a need for any such expertise consult with the appropriate professional. This book does not contain all information available on the subject. This book has not been created to be specific to any individual's or organizations' situation or needs. Every effort has been made to make this book as accurate as possible. However, there may be typographical and or content errors. Therefore, this book should serve only as a general guide and not as the ultimate source of subject information. This book contains information that might be dated and is intended only to educate and entertain. The author and publisher shall have no liability or responsibility to any person or entity regarding any loss or damage incurred, or alleged to have incurred, directly or indirectly, by the information contained in this book.

DEDICATION

To all those fighting a battle of your own, and to the families that work so hard yet struggle to help. This is for you!

Paul, my Penguin. You loved me when I couldn't love myself. You persevered, knocked down my walls and took the time to build me back up piece by piece with your unconditional love. You are the reason I became the person I am proud to be today. Thank you for motivating me to write my story.

Thank you for your friendship, **Marlena**. Your inspirational story touched my heart. You have overcome so much in your life and showed me what strength really is. I took from this whenever I was faced with moments of hesitation and doubt.

My life forever changed when I met you, **Karli**. I was drawn to you for a reason and believe that we crossed paths at a time that I needed it most. You are an incredibly special person and will always have a special place in my heart. Love you more than chocolate!

Elaine, you were the first person I trusted with my secret. You listened without judgement and encouraged me to put my feelings to paper. Thank you for being so easy to talk to.

ACKNOWLEDGMENTS

Kat, you were the roadmap to making my story come to light. You were the glue that brought it all together. Thank you for helping me dig deep and get over the finish line.

ABOUT THE AUTHOR

Shani grew up in Newcastle, England with childhood secrets
that manifested into a battle with Bulimia.

She emigrated to Arizona, where she started to unpeel the
complex layers of emotions that her secrets had inflicted. As
she incorporated life changing habits into her lifestyle, she
was able to heal and overcome her turbulent and dangerous
relationship with her eating disorder.

Writing was always just a therapeutic outlet until
she realized she had something valuable to share. Turning
her own journey of self-help into a path to help others, is
how War with Myself was born.

CONTENTS

1

JOURNEY INTO HELL

When I was a young child in England, in a confusing and difficult world, I didn't know at the time, but a courtship had started with an unseen enemy, fierce and formidable. It would take me years to realize that I was dancing a strange but alluring dance with a powerful entity that was hell bent on leading me into a deep darkness.

This enemy captivated and intoxicated me, weaving its spell and tethering me with such weighted chains that escape seemed futile. I didn't know for some time that I was on a path of self-destruction.

I didn't know I'd be living in hell on earth.

*L*et me explain. You see, the enemy was bulimia nervosa. This pernicious and complicated eating disorder does not discriminate between gender, ethnicity or how much money you have. It most often afflicts women, but men have also fallen prey. In the US alone, 1.5 percent of women or 4.7 million, develop bulimia while only 0.5 percent are men. Unfortunately, in the UK and around the world, eating disorders have become a prevalent problem. Bulimia is often characterized by binge eating, often with high caloric foods and then purging. The act of release. The malady, if not stopped, can be life threatening with a life expectancy of about 15 years.

Eating disorders may first manifest during adolescent years and are more common in 18 to 35-year-olds. Although sadly, there have been cases found in children as young as 6 or in people as old as 70. With Bulimia, the average age of onset is 18-19 years of age.

I can attest to that. I was 20 when bulimia fully engaged. Yet, the foundation was laid when I was just a little girl. My world, and my family were in freefall.

I was born in the Northeast of England in one of the most iconic cities in Britain, Newcastle-upon-Tyne. It is now most commonly referred to as Newcastle and boasts jaw dropping architecture and is full of history. I remember, even from a young age, the city centre was remarkably busy and fast paced with an infectious happy vibe. People were always moving, doing something.

Newcastle used to be a coal mining town and was a major shipbuilding and manufacturing hub. Over the years it has grown into a popular destination due to becoming the centre of business, arts, and sciences.

As a child, my family lived on the outskirts of all that beauty, in a two-story council house nestled in what you'd call a rough estate. Council houses were established in 1919 right after the end of World War I.

They provided desperately needed housing for soldiers and their families. The tradition continues today, which helps families similar to mine, have a decent roof over their heads when they can't otherwise afford to live without government subsidy. My mum and dad, three brothers, my sister and I lived on the corner of our cul-de-sac on Apsley Crescent, with blueberry bushes that separated our home from the street. On the other side of the road was a big field that over-looked a huge park that was surrounded by lush green trees. This was often the place I'd go to, to feel free, have fun and just be a kid.

Both of my parents were supported by the government. But my dad would always do odd jobs for people and get paid under the table. We weren't a close-knit family. We didn't play games, have designated family time, or even eat together. We were just there, often playing with our toys, keeping each other occupied or watching cartoons on tv. My parents were incredibly young, and this contributed to their parenting style. We didn't know any different. We enjoyed the life we had. I don't really remember my dad being home much during those earlier years. He was out a lot and wasn't what you'd call a present father. He was either galivanting with friends, visiting his mum, gambling at the betting shop with what little money we had or sneaking around with other girls, although I didn't know this at the time.

My mum often speaks of her courtship with my dad with high regard and with smiles that would light up her face. She said he was always affectionate and treated her very well. They were so happy in love and were always together. But over time, his personality started changing and his patience grew shorter along with his temper. It was never directed at us kids. He would fly off the handle and shout at us when he was angry about something but never abusive towards us.

He'd smack us if we were naughty but back then it wasn't a big deal. His attacks were always targeted towards Mum. He became verbally abusive if she said or did something he didn't like. Then the emotional abuse would escalate to physical beatings. He would push her around and it progressed to backhanding her across the face and would twist her arm behind her back, almost breaking it.

The emotional turmoil mixed with the physical pain must have been so much to endure. Me being the eldest, I could feel the tension during those times. She'd try her hardest to hide everything from us and would keep her feelings and emotions locked up inside. She was brave and had such a strong exterior. No-one would have known anything other than what was portrayed, a happy marriage.

It got so bad that my mum tried to leave several times. The police were called and they snuck us off to a hostel for battered women. I loved it. It was like staying in a hotel. I had other kids to play with. It was like going on holiday. I didn't want to go back home.

Dad would always figure out where we were and would convince my mum that he was sorry and that he would never do it again. He would beg her to take him back. And of course, she did. I hated that she would fall for it. It never changed.

My dad suffered from migraines and used to take Solpadeine, dissolvable pills that were sold over the counter. It wasn't until years later that it became known that they were highly addictive. He'd eat them like sweets throughout the day and gradually took so much that he'd have to purchase them from different chemists as they became more controlled. So, I'm fairly sure it was this that caused the changes within him. Knowing what I do now, it makes it easier to understand him and how he was back then.

It's weird. I don't remember feeling terribly negative towards my dad. I loved him. It was more of a feeling in the household, like heavy air. I knew some of what was happening, and it made me anxious, although I didn't know how to explain the uneasy feeling at the time. It was then that I started to fidget by rubbing material between my thumb and finger. It felt so good, it had a calming effect. I would do it so often that I would end up putting holes in the fabric. As an adult I found out that it was a self-soothing mechanism to distract from negative feelings caused by anxiety and stress. I still do it now when I have something on my mind. Anxiety plays a major part in eating disorders.

Fundamentally, anxiety is a normal reaction to anything stressful that pushes the person to act in a situation that may be harmful. It can be a life-saving reaction, but often it can get out of control. It is one of the most prevalent mental health disorders today.

The problem gets bad when you begin to get distressed and worry about everything, even insignificant things. I began to realize that I was having anxious moments. One incident in particular always caused anxiety. Even looking back at it now, it still bothers me.

We'd often visit someone. I don't know who it was, but I remember there being a side door with a tiny square porch where a young man would 'play' with me. He'd sit down with his back against the wall and sit me on his lap pretending that I'd be riding a horse. He'd bounce me up and down on his lap like I was galloping and would use sound effects as he'd rub himself against me. It wasn't until I was old enough to comprehend this that I realized what 'play' really meant to him.

Whenever I think about this, his face is blurred out of my memory.I'm not sure why. However, I always think about my Auntie's ex-husband. The thought is always there with nothing to back it up. My mum later told me that there were rumors that he was a pedophile. His children want nothing to do with him. I'm unsure if this has anything to do with it as we have never spoken about this and never will do. It corroborates my gut feeling, but it's certainly not proof, and will always be something I question.

Well, things continued to deteriorate with my mum and dad.

My mum was friends with a lady who lived up the street from us.

After a while, she also became friends with her husband, Al. My mum started to confide in him and eventually, they started an emotional affair and crafted a getaway plan. Cases were packed and under the bed waiting for the right time. One day when my dad was out visiting his mum, we all left on a cold snowy day, oblivious as to what was taking place.

We walked to the metro station and got off in town. Then Al, his son Micah, my four siblings, my mum and I got on a Greyhound bus from Newcastle to Walsall. Nine hours later we arrived at my Nana's house.

Living with my Nana was fun. We hadn't seen her in so long. Due to limited space, some of us kids had to share a double bed. But we didn't care.

This is when my childhood innocence came to a halt, and my future of protecting Micah who was about 14, began. I didn't really understand what was going on at the time. Who would at 9? When it started, he was so nonchalant. He'd check that the door was closed and that no one was around, which is how I sensed that something wasn't quite right. He told me to pull down my knickers and guided me into the position he wanted me in, which was lying flat with my legs over the side of the bed, so my bottom was on the edge.

He tried to put his penis inside of me. When it didn't work, he climbed on top of me and started rubbing himself against me. The warmth of his breath felt uncomfortable on the side of my face and the grunting sounds he made will forever stay with me. I just stayed still, somehow unable to move until he was finished.

I'd be red afterwards because of the friction. When he was done, he'd pull up his trousers and I'd do the same. Then we'd both get on with our day. Never talking about it.

I never said no. I didn't really understand what I was supposed to be saying no to. One day Mum walked into the bedroom to find Micah on top of me. She was shocked and started screaming frantically and smacked him across the face. Al came barging in and told us both to go downstairs.

He beat him. Micah said that he was sorry and cried out that he wanted to move back to Newcastle with his mum. They thought that was that.

I don't remember any conversations or questions about if it had happened before, or when it started or how I felt about it. Nothing. They just assumed that it was dealt with, and it was never mentioned again. Whenever anything happened, it was like that particular moment was frozen in time. And for some reason I was able to disconnect and allow it to happen. That was until I was older and started to understand and feelings started to emerge.

Dad was furious that my mum had left and taken the kids with her. So much so that he came to Walsall and kidnapped my biological brothers Michael and Peter when they were playing out in the front garden. This caused a lot of stress in the household and it would be a while before they were back home with us and everything was back to normal. To make things easier, we moved back to Newcastle.

My dad ended up remarried to a woman that obviously didn't like having us around. We threatened her new family. I tried so hard to have a relationship with him. I longed for his love and attention. I didn't want to disrupt his life. Just be a part of it.

Over the years, as I was becoming more aware of what was happening with Micah, I became more confused about how I felt.

Yet, I still did nothing to stop it. During my early teens when I was having major Daddy issues, it was obvious that what I was experiencing was wrong. This led to increased anxiety. I started avoiding Micah as I was scared to be alone with him. This was about the time that my eating habits started to change. I was feeling like I was losing control.

I'd send my dad letters begging him to see me. I'd find out where he lived and just turn up. Quite often, he'd leave shortly after I arrived. He didn't care, or at least that's how he acted.

I confided in a social worker to try and work through my tumultuous emotions. I had a solicitor to communicate with my dad as a mediator. Mum was so angry with him as she could see the pain I was in, and she felt helpless. I was so emotional. I'd cry all the time.

My mum is only 15 years older than me. We weren't close and I fought with her a lot in my teenage years which is why she helped me to get my own flat at 16. But I have to take my hat off to her as, during these trying times with my dad, she was my rock and she advocated for me as much as any person could.

It hurt so much to know that I was putting in all this effort and my own dad couldn't care less about me. What makes a father turn away from his daughter? It's unnatural.

The utter pain of his rejection tore through my heart like a razor blade, leaving a void that couldn't be filled. Perhaps, later on, I tried to fill that void with food. Was I unlovable? I may have thought so at the time. Rejection from a parent is a torturous thing.

Parents are supposed to love us regardless of what we do. The problem was, and still is, that we can't go back and undo the hurts. There are no do-overs. If a parent doesn't love you, how can someone else? How can you love yourself? That's the biggest issue that leads to our devaluation, and often to our destruction.

2

BULLIES, BOOZE AND...

On the verge of an eating disorder, you often are unaware about what is happening to you. Things seem to spiral out of control and suddenly you discover yourself in the strong grip of something overpowering. Back then, the idea that an eating disorder was manifesting ready to hijack my wellbeing, wasn't even on my radar.

With so much going on in your brain, you're too busy fending off swarms of emotional mosquitos that slowly extract pieces of you. A switch seems to be flipped that leads a person down an ominous path. It doesn't matter if the switch was done so by something internal or external. Although I would say that external components were very much a part of my problem.

At about 12, I was in high school. By then, I was skipping breakfast. I'd eat at lunch and then I would barely touch anything in the evening. If I did, I would pick and move food around the plate, so that it looked like I had eaten. Anything to keep my mum off my back.

Honestly, I often didn't feel hungry at all. I was so slim that people would comment at school all the time. They weren't nice comments either. Bean pole or lamp post was a popular barb. My peers thought it was funny to tell Ethiopian jokes, or say I looked like a golf club. A boy that liked me even told me that he'd seen better legs on a coffee table. I always laughed it off. Never showing how hurtful it really was. At that age, children are so sensitive about appearances and of course, anyone who doesn't look like the rest of the crowd is singled out.

This was the beginning of the foundational cracks in my self-esteem. Hearing all these negative things every day certainly took a toll on my emotional wellbeing.

On top of everything, when I got home, my mum would be waiting for me. She would tell me I needed to eat more. I wasn't allowed to leave the kitchen until I was done. Sometimes she'd wait so long that she would get frustrated and try to force feed me. It didn't work. It just made me gag. All her attempts had the opposite effect. As her concerns grew, so did my rebellious nature. It would cause arguments and tension would begin to build.

I ended up at the Nuffield Hospital as an outpatient where I saw doctors and nutritionists. During this time, my school life took a turn when the name calling evolved to bullying. The escalation was horrific, and I sensed it was going to get uglier.

Suddenly it was like there was a spotlight on me. It was a free for all. There was a girl, Julie. I will never forget her. I remember her big round head with such tight red curls and a sinister grin that is deeply etched into my memory. Her reputation would precede her. Hearing her name was enough to make me hold my breath and make me cringe.

Although she herself did nothing to me physically, she had many minions that would be only too happy to do her dirty work. There was no reason behind why it started. It just did. One day I walked by her group of friends, and she pushed one of them into me. She then acted like I'd bumped into her on purpose and started talking all tough and saying I pushed her.

She looked back to the group and of course they were fueling her fire. Chanting "Go on hit her! She pushed you so she's looking for a fight."

She pushed me around a few times as I stumbled. I stood back up and tried to pull myself together. I managed to walk away. After that day, it became more often. I tried to find alternate routes, stay away from the girl's toilets and would be vigilant on my way to class.

Then, I would have girls saying that I should watch my back and that so-and-so was going to be waiting for me after school. I never knew any of these girls. As I left the school grounds, sure enough, there they were. There were 6-8 of them huddled together with smirks on their faces. They towered over me. My heart pounded so hard. I was in disbelief that people I did not know would go to such lengths to make my school life miserable. The first time I was jumped on I was left bruised, shaken, confused and with an imprint of a sovereign ring on my forehead and bloody scratches. The imprint of the ring lasted for a couple of weeks. I was branded. Plain and simple.

Luckily, I had long hair. My fringe was always tied up in my ponytail, but after this incident I wore my hair down to the side in order to hide it. When the scabs had healed a bit and the bruising turned yellow, it was harder to tell what it was. Just a bruise. It looked like I just banged it.

I was jumped on periodically until I was 16, which is when school ended back then in England. I couldn't even feel safe walking the streets of where I lived since the bullying overflowed to my homelife.

One day I was walking up the street and two girls asked me the time. I said, "Sorry, but I don't have a watch." So, I didn't know. They jumped me, dragged me by my hair and repeatedly slammed my head against the concrete path. The whole ordeal was extremely aggressive and was especially traumatic.

The layers of hurt continued to grow day by day. And as time went by, I was stripped of the person I was, to make way for the person I'd become. Someone I didn't know.

The bullying pushed me to the very brink. Bullying, especially when it concerns how a person looks, triggers a waterfall of emotions and distress. According to the National Eating Disorder Association, 65 percent of the people who have developed eating disorders believe that bullying may have been the cause.

Most people are unaware of the prevalence of bullying and the damage it can do to someone, especially children. In America, 10 million males alone, have eating disorders founded in bullying. It's a social phenomenon tearing through schools and hearts leaving a path of destruction in its wake. In children who are overweight, 40 percent of them have eating disorders.

A coldness and a negativity take root in people subject to bullying. A strong fear develops in those that are bullied to the extent that life looks bleak. It was during my experience with bullies that I first had overwhelming negative thoughts. They would flow over me like a tidal wave ready to take away my pain. When I would wait for traffic, I'd look out to the cars and imagine myself walking in front of them. It would be easy. It would all be over. No one would care.

I'd also think about survival. What if I did this and I survived with major injuries, or were in a vegetative state, or were paralyzed? I couldn't bear that. I'd rather it be over quickly. I'd think about the ways that I could end my life that would hurt the least.

The high mortality rate in people with eating disorders is from suicide and not from their compromised physical condition. Additionally, according to the University of Minnesota Psychiatric Department, bulimics and those suffering from purging disorders are at higher risk for suicide. Interesting to note, eating disorders and suicide attempts run in families.

In my family, my youngest sister slit her wrists and fortunately survived. Being overwhelmed and not seeing an end to her physical and emotional pain was just too much for her to bear at her young age. My brother was and had been severely depressed, which led to him hanging himself. Luckily, it was unsuccessful, and he survived. My mum battled with her own demons with depression and suicidal thoughts too. As for me, I didn't really *want* to die. I just wanted all the bad stuff to end. Granted, suicide may seem like the solution, but it really isn't.

It's amazing how pushed we can be when under duress and desperate to stop the pain. We think killing ourselves is the answer. I'm so grateful that I grew up in a time where there was no social media. I don't want to think about how things might have been different if social media was as popular back then as it is now.

Of course, no one knew what was happening in my day-to-day life. No one then could step up to help me. I was still dealing with Micah and trying to stay afloat. I was also feeling worthless, unloved, and unwanted because my own dad didn't want anything to do with me. The emotional toll it took on me was grueling. I would cry so hard and long in private that my chest would hurt, my face would swell up and my jaw would ache. It contributed to me losing my appetite. Science has discovered that anorexia is not only a psychiatric disorder but that it also has components of a metabolic disorder and can be discovered in genome mapping. It wasn't known at the time I was going through all of this. To be honest, even if it were, my family wouldn't have known to test for it.

I became more withdrawn at school. I didn't do anything at all to defend myself. I hated myself for that. As time passed, my schoolwork suffered due to me not reaching out when I needed help. I didn't want to bring attention to myself in class. I found it harder to concentrate and retain information. Some of that was down to lack of nutrients. I was once a good student and enjoyed school, but that quickly declined.

Sometimes I'd feel like I wasn't in my own body. Sometimes I'd feel like I was living in slow motion. My brain was foggy at times too. It was a hit and miss with food. I was still eating when I had an appetite, but it was common for me to skip meals or multiple meals a day. I never really tracked it, but I wonder if there was a correlation between how much stress I was under and the food I consumed during that period.

I'd find myself sitting with my head in my hands feeling confused as to why I was going through this. Why me? What did I do to make so many people hate me? Still feeling like my mum was overacting with the food because, I was still eating.

The overall stress of everything in my school life and at home would impact my sleep. There were nights when I'd be lying awake for hours tossing and turning. When I finally dozed off, I'd have bad dreams and would often wake up with cold sweats. As I got older and was battling with Bulimia, my anxiety dreams were worse, recurring, and vivid. It would be safe to assume I was also suffering from PTSD.

I remember I started to get constipated in my early teens. It was because I wasn't eating properly. I'd get pains in my stomach that were so excruciating, I thought that something could be seriously wrong. When I felt really anxious, I got diarrhea. These were all early signs that my body was trying to tell me that something wasn't right.

It is common for people with eating disorders to look in the mirror often with a most critical eye. I actually didn't look in the mirror a lot in my teen years. I didn't wear makeup and hadn't really noticed myself in any way negative or positive.

There were no negative feelings to the way I looked at all. I often questioned if I was ugly because of how I was being treated. Not that that would have been a good reason. I couldn't get past that there was just no reason for it at all.

I didn't open up to the doctors or nurses about what was going on with me. I kept it to myself. What friends I had didn't do anything about the bullying. Nor did we talk about it. They were scared for themselves. I never talked to my friends about home life either.

I was supposed to talk about my eating habits at the hospital. Nothing stuck as I didn't have a problem with food itself. I wasn't scared of putting on weight. I would have quite liked to put weight on at the time. It was solely loss of appetite. I wasn't purposefully restricting food intake. I had no interest in food whatsoever.

Looking back and knowing what I do now, I would say that I was anorexic. I didn't know what it was back then. Not for a long time. Even as I got older and became more educated on the subject, I assumed you had to deprive yourself of every meal to be diagnosed with anorexia.

Things deteriorated. I lived every day looking over my shoulder. In a constant state of dread, and in anticipation of the unknown. I lived with the embarrassment of knowing that people at school saw what was happening. The fear of the physical pain and the torment of the emotional pain was tremendous. With everything that I was going through, self-loathing soon took its hold on me.

I was embarrassed and ashamed that I didn't do anything about it. I didn't defend myself until the last few weeks of school when a boy pushed in front of me in the lunch queue as people always did. I said, "There's a line you know," with an attitude.

He asked, "What you going to do about it?"

I responded with an impactful punch in the face. Not a good response, I know. But it made me feel good at the time.

Eventually I told my mum about some of the bullying. She talked to the headmaster. The headmaster's response was that I was not a good student because my grades had declined. So, he was inclined to believe the stories of others in the class.

They said that I was disruptive and made it hard for them to concentrate. He added that I didn't do my portion of the assignments when we were asked to work as a group. He didn't believe that they wouldn't *allow* me to participate. He also brought up that I was skipping classes. I was. It got so bad that some classes would cause me so much anxiety that I just couldn't go any more. I'd never been sent to the head-master office before and now I was labeled as a bad student.

He didn't want to hear my side of the story. So, nothing changed. Only now, they made fun of me because in their words, I went running to mummy.

My homelife was in an uproar and my mother and I were not getting along. She was still in a relationship with Al. One night we were playing monopoly. Others had gone bankrupt and went to their room. I was still in the game but was eager for it to be over after an hour. Al would get annoyed at the smallest things, and he would say, "Don't start a game if you can't finish it." I didn't want him to get angry, so I stayed.

I looked at his drink that he had been sipping on during the game. "Oooh orange juice!" I could just use a drink. So, I asked if I could have a sip. He said yes. It tasted a little off, but some cheap brands taste different, so I didn't think anything of it. He smiled and asked if I wanted some more. I was thirsty and it was a nice break from the game, so I drank up until the glass was empty.

He left to go refill his drink. Only a little amount of time had gone by when I started to feel a little dizzy, like the room was spinning. Al laughed and told me there was vodka in the orange juice. He found it funny that I was drunk. I quickly stumbled up the stairs and went to bed. As I lay the room was spinning and I felt so nauseous.

My mum was furious and worried in case I choked on my vomit in the night. Eventually I fell asleep as she stroked my hair and we never brought it up again.

Other things materialized. When I was about fourteen, one night, my mum went to bed, and I stayed up watching TV with Al. The lights were off, so it was dark in the sitting room, and you could see the lights flickering on the walls. I was curled up all cozy on the settee. He was flicking through the channels and when he stopped, he sat back and relaxed into the chair. I soon realized that this was a soft porn movie. I didn't know what to do. Should I watch, should I turn away? Then I thought about how sick it was that he was watching this whilst I was in the room. I froze and was too scared to move. After what felt like forever, I managed to pluck up the courage to get up and go to bed.

Even though there was no abuse from Al, he made me feel uncomfortable to be alone with him and believe he should never have put me in those situations. They have stuck with me over the years.

As for Micah it was easier to see where he might have gotten some of his ideas with Al's penchant for porn. I was in my early teens, and one of our encounters was different. Usually when it was happening, I'd lay there until he was done and then we'd both go our separate ways. This time, there was a sensation I'd never felt before. It tingled and felt warm. I couldn't explain it. But I liked it.

When he was done, I was still. I was numb. Then I'd have an emotional feeling that I didn't know how to describe. At this age, I knew this was wrong, but I never stopped him or told anyone. I allowed it. I never once spoke to him about it, nor did he with me, ever.

I quickly realized that the emotions I was feeling were disgust and shame. Disgusted that I never said no, and ashamed that I liked it. How sick am I? I was so confused.

Micah and I had always seemed like we got on. But suddenly, I found myself picking fights with him. I'd get him into trouble on purpose. He'd annoy me, and I'd make it known. I was spiteful and I didn't care. It was my way of getting back at him in any way I knew how. He was older than I and he took advantage of me.

When I was young and innocent, I had no idea what he was doing. He robbed me of many things, including my dignity. Without a doubt, those encounters brought me to a precipice.

3

REBORN

Breaking free from the chains that bound me to my pain was like a Phoenix rising from the ashes. When I graduated high school at 16, I was free from the bullies.

I soared high above the anguish and all the moments that haunted me as I moved out, and at last was mature enough to better cope with the dynamic of the forced one-sided relationship with my dad.

The first link in the chain broke at 14 when I begged my mum to let me stay with my nana and Auntie Maureen.

Maureen was mentally handicapped, and Nana was her full-time care giver. I was so excited when she said yes. It was only temporary, but I didn't care. All I could think about was that I had my own room. It was a stress-free environment, which contributed to an increase in my appetite.

I was more relaxed than I had ever remembered. This helped me to recoup after a hard day at school. I was happy and grateful that there were no encounters with Micah during or after this time.

Establishing my own place helped give me a sense of freedom from the trauma and the distress that my family home haunted me with.

At 16, I was approved to get a government subsidized one bedroom flat. It wasn't in the best of areas, but it could have been much worse. It was mine. The government provided a care package that included a bed, wardrobe, kitchen ware and a decorating allowance, which helped kick start my new life.

It was close enough to my family that I could visit as often as I liked. The government would review my paycheck on a weekly basis and would subsidize my income accordingly, so that I always had enough to live on.

It was an especially exciting time for me. Although, the elation was short-lived.

A few months after I settled into my new home, I learned that Micah and his girlfriend moved into the flats that joined mine. So much for freedom and security.

This made me uncomfortable. It was like a dark cloud looming over me. I didn't see him too often, but when I did, we acted *Normal*. Well, my memories were there, memories of lost innocence and tumult. I tried to work through it, but I stuffed my emotions down deep.

The scars from earlier years were not yet healed. How else was I supposed to act if I didn't want to disrupt the status quo and cause tension that others could feel and question? I was in control now. And for me, that meant keeping the feelings he evoked in check.

I had my flat for about a year before they were demolished, in an effort to rebuild and enhance the estate. My only option was to move back in with my family. At the time, I worked at a ladies' only gym. I worked in sales and helped on the gym floor, assisting with the introductory sessions. I was simultaneously taking classes in business and customer service at the local community college. I enjoyed the work and it kept me busy. I was starting to feel like things were on track.

In a way, my day-to-day life allowed me to learn more about who I was. Not really feeling authentically happy, I struggled, and it was often a tug of war with my inner self. It was a time of exploration as it was for many girls my age. My need to find myself was reaching critical mass.

Soon after I celebrated my 19th birthday, I went on a trip to Spain with my brothers' girlfriend, Victoria. We decided that it would be fun to pretend to be different people. So, we invented alter egos. We produced different names and concocted stories about who we were and what we did for work.

It was fun to play someone other than myself for a change. My new name was to be Shani for the duration of the trip. My real name was Valerie. A lot of baggage came with that name, and I was glad to shed it. Little did I know that my temporary personality was more the real me than I realized. It was the part of me I had to hide away. The excitable me that had been waiting to burst out, waiting to shine.

The energy in Spain was electric. I felt alive for the first time. Severed from the shackles of Valerie and all that she represented; I was gloriously distracted from the reminder that I was never enough, not enough for my dad, for people at school, nor for John.

I should introduce you to John, my first boyfriend.

He was significant in my life from 15-17 and was the first person I had met that didn't want anything from me. John was the first person that showed me true kindness. He earned my trust. We had known each other back when we were kids playing in the local YMCA.

Our first date was walking around Newcastle City Centre. The Big Market is a particular area in town where streets are filled with people bobbing and weaving through the weekend market stalls, but at night it turned into one of the most popular destinations for night life.

I remember the hustle and bustle of the crowds, the smell of the restaurant food in the air and the music blaring from the bars nearby like it was yesterday. It was magical. We ended the day eating at KFC where he had me try his favorite burger, the Zinger burger. I still love it today.

During the beginning of our relationship was when my anxiety dreams regarding sex were at the highest. I was so scared that he'd try something for which I was not ready. I was particularly good at hiding the anguish it caused. But soon, he showed me that everything was in my own time. He never tried anything or crossed any line. I felt like he was following my lead, and that felt good. I could relax.

When I was with him, I felt better about myself. He gave me the strength to cope with school as I finally had some light in my life and a reason to go on.

He paved the way for me to open myself up to others. Amazingly, he allowed me to see that not everyone had an agenda. I didn't have to be afraid of the unknown. In fact, I could trust others, even though it didn't always work out. He showed me that it was worth trying.

I never told him about Micah, but I openly talked about other unwanted situations that I found myself in.

It broke my heart to let him go. The day we sat on the green and he explained how he wanted to "play the field" was a memory that was bittersweet. We were both so young and he didn't want us to stay together and grow apart, or later have regrets. He was so honest, and I could tell it genuinely pained him to say those words.

The last thing he wanted to do was hurt me. He held me tightly as we both shed tears and lingered as we said our goodbyes. I walked away with an aching in my heart I had never felt before. This was the moment when I understood the term *heartbreak*. I had to be brave if I wanted him in my life. Even if it was just as friends. Although it was hard in the beginning, we stayed in contact and even today we talk with very fond memories.

I met John for a reason. He was to be in my life when I thought there was no life to have. He was my lifeline. Being with him allowed me to close a wound, open up my heart and build enough trust to feel safe. Our relationship was the foundation to future relationships.

It was on my trip to Spain that I met Karli. Victoria and I needed space. She was a negative person that sucked my energy. I definitely didn't need that. I met Karli in the lobby of the hotel. She was stunning and stood out, with her amazing figure. Karli had short dyed red hair, and a contagious laugh. Every person we walked past would take a second look.

From the second I met her, we clicked. It felt like I had always known her. We talked for hours at the local bars, got a little tipsy, ok well a lot tipsy and did some embarrassing stuff we would laugh about for years, even to this day. Things like skinny dipping and singing fun songs at the top of our voices in the streets like we didn't have a care in the world. I felt so free spirited when I was around her. We would laugh so hard our tummies would hurt, but we could have more meaningful conversations, too. She had an energy that drew me in. I loved being around her.

Soon I realized that people really liked my persona I had in Spain. They wanted to hang out. They treated me with respect. I liked this person too. I smiled all the time. I laughed so hard at times I'd cry. I connected with someone on a genuine level not knowing that she'd become my life-long friend. It was such a breath of fresh air. When I realized that it was truly me on holiday and not just a person I made up, I decided to do something that would change my life forever.

When I got home from Spain, I talked to my mum about how she would feel if I were to change my name. Afterall, I was named after her. Surprisingly, she was supportive and urged me to do what I felt was right for me, and not to worry about anyone else's opinion. We talked about hyphenating my name. She liked the idea, and it was nice that she had some involvement in the change. A few days later I went to a solicitor's office and changed my name legally. Goodbye Valerie and the pain that held on to her and hello Shani-Lee, the happy, gregarious person that was eager to be reborn.

4

DANCING TO A NEW BEAT

"I AM HERE." My inner self clawed her way to the forefront eager to be seen and heard after so many years of being suppressed. I felt amazing.

I'd only been home for a few weeks when Karli and I talked about what we wanted out of life. All we were sure of is that we wanted life experiences and the personal growth that came along with that.

We were going with the flow and the flow wasn't in a direction we necessarily wanted. We decided that we were just going to pack up and move to the place that brought us together and inspired us. Spain.

We didn't have a job or anywhere to stay lined up. We just assumed that it would work itself out. We had nothing to lose. Within a month we had both quit our jobs and off we went.

As soon as we arrived, we went to a night club that we frequented whilst on holiday. We had previously met the owner. He recognized us and gave us both a job as go-go dancers. Our job was to motivate people to get up and dance and have a good time. We could do that. We loved to dance. He also had a friend that had an oceanfront apartment that would become available in a few days.

We stayed in a hostel until it was ready. Before we knew it, we were a part of the holiday lifestyle in Magaluf Majorca, one of the hottest holiday destinations at the time. It was one of the most memorable times of my life. I'm so grateful that I got to experience it with Karli.

Living in Spain was tiring but filled with fun. We worked from 11pm-6am. When we finally got used to working at night and we no longer had whiplash and sore bodies from all the dancing we would do on a nightly basis, we started to enjoy our time more. We'd meet at a local bar with other workers. This was like our happy hour. We'd go to the beach, shop in the markets, enjoy jeep drives through the mountains and go to parties. There was one that was particularly memorable.

Karli and I had met some guys at a bar who managed a yacht. It was christened, Kymet. They said they liked the fact that we were down to earth and enjoyed spending time with us. It was nothing more than just friends.

Once we got to know them, they invited us to a boat party. They told us the theme was, black and white, and said they would pick us up.

We thought why not? By that time, we were allowed one night off a week, so we might as well make the most of it. We had our outfits all planned out. Karli wore a psychedelic looking black and white mini dress. Mine was a white lace dress that my skin peered through. We both felt incredible and were ready for some fun on the water.

The guys pulled up in a red sporty Porsche. We jumped in and off we went. Karli and I looked confused as we pulled up. We had passed the marina. We got out and walked down an archway that was beautifully manicured with green vines and pretty flowers. We entered a building with cathedral ceilings and gigantic crystal chandeliers that glistened in the light.

Karli and I smiled at the grandeur of it all, but still confused as we were told it was a *boat* party. Well, it was a free night out with some guys that made us laugh. We shrugged our shoulders and we all continued to walk towards the music with huge smiles, excited for the night ahead.

When we opened the double doors, my eyes widened, and my heart jumped. I stared at Karli, then looked at the guys and I think I swore. In fact, I know I did. It was a very stately ball room with marble everywhere. On the floors, going up the pillars to the ceiling, it had the biggest multi layered chandelier I've ever seen. There was a live band on the stage that was more like an orchestra with a singer. People were in tuxedos and the women were in black and white ball gowns.

The guys could see we were in disbelief. They ushered us to our designated table and on the way, we passed the elaborate over the top catered tables. I stopped when I saw a pig with an apple in its mouth and hooves that were displayed around it. I'd never seen anything like it.

When we got to our table it was a mixture of laughing with nervous energy and questions that we had spewed out. Our initial thought was that they done it to embarrass us. But why? We stood out like a sore thumb. There was no way that this was a mistake.

They told us that the reason they invited us was because we were a breath of fresh air compared to all the pretentious people they were often around. They wanted *us* to attend the ball and not some made up version of us. When they told us that it was a boat party, it was us who misunderstood.

It was an event for those that *owned* boats. Yachts to be precise. Once the explanations were out of the way, we decided to make the most of it and have some fun.

The room was filled with people that were high up in society and snobbish. The women gave us dirty looks but after we started dancing and being ourselves, we found that some of the men that were in attendance were asking us to dance and were eager to join in on the fun we were obviously having.

It turned out to be an amazing and memorable night. As we left the 'boat party' we ran down the hallway with our heels in our hands laughing at what had just transpired. It was certainly a night to remember.

There were so many amazing memories I took away from Spain, all locked up in my memory bank for a rainy day. Yet, they weren't tucked away too snugly. I was always ready to take them out and reminisce when Karli and I would meet for a cup of tea and a catch up.

It wasn't the only thing I brought back with me. With a combination of free drinks and a staple diet of pasta and sandwiches, it wasn't surprising that I put on some weight. Others noticed and commented, which was hurtful. But it wasn't something about which I was concerned.

I moved to Stratford-upon-Avon as soon as I got back from Spain. It was a beautiful historic town where William Shakespeare lived. The Tudor houses, blooming flowers, scenic canals with waterfront theaters and cultural attractions made it a perfect picturesque place to live.

My relationship with my mum was much better. We stayed connected, and she would keep me updated on how my siblings were doing. During one of our calls, my mum's voice was a little shaky. When I asked what was wrong, she told me that my Aunt Maureen had been raped and was pregnant.

My initial thought went straight to Micah. I had no evidence to base this off. It was just my experience and the fact that he would visit sometimes and would stay even if Nana weren't there. I felt sick at the thought that someone would do this to a mentally handicapped person, with the emotional age of five.

I also felt torn about whether I should say something or not. If I did, they would surely want to know the reasoning behind this. It wasn't something I was ready to talk about. Even though I had moved away and was no longer in contact with Micah, I knew that he was still in contact with the rest of the family.

Guilt overtook me for a long time. I knew that I could have some information that could help answer my family's questions, but I was confused. It may not have been him. I may have just been biased. It wasn't until years later when I told my mum that she allowed me to release what I was holding on to and move on from the guilt.

At 20, I ended up moving to Leamington Spa for a job in a gym and to be closer to Karli. I was putting myself through college again. This time in Media Production and Marketing. I also did contract work with a marketing company. It was stressful to do everything with no family support. But life was good.

Karli's parents helped me more than they could ever know. My heart boasts with the respect and love I have for them. In a time of need, when my own family was unable to be there, Lynn and Phil were my parents. They invited me into their home anytime I needed a place to stay or just to visit. They supported me and checked in to make sure I was ok. Healthy positive relationships were not a staple part of my childhood. I had to find these relationships on my own, starting with Karli and her family.

5

THORNS AMONG THE ROSES

If you're lucky, certain moments in your life lead you to fulfillment and to love, but sadly, we often fail to recognize the crossroads that lie before us and may take the wrong path. We are too busy or too preoccupied to notice. In a rush, the road signs blur or we miss them entirely. So, we don't know that we've missed our turn. Yet, fate has a way of pulling us from our detours.

Paul was the best friend of my boss, John. He was English but his work as an Engineer took him to Germany where he lived. He would come to visit John whenever he was in town and would often take the time to talk to me. He was 10 years older than me, had a stable career and knew what he wanted in life. His temperament was calming. There was something special about him. We'd become good friends over time. In our conversations, he had always said that he never wanted to get married or have kids. We'd laugh about it, but he was serious. We became friends of the moment, only talking when he was in town visiting John.

Then, there was Bryan. I'd see Bryan every time he came into the gym. The duration of our conversations got longer and longer. He was a few years older and was from Michigan. He was also an Engineer and was working in England for a few months. He seemed different to other guys. He was quiet, reserved, and shy. He was almost gentle with me. Since he didn't know anyone except for work colleagues, we spent time together. It was easy. He made me laugh.

I loved to hear stories about his life. His time in a Fraternity was especially intriguing. It was so foreign to me. We slowly became more than just friends with the understanding that it would end when he went back home to the US. Our first date was amazing. One of our earlier conversations was about the differences in the US vs England.

At the time, we didn't have high school proms and so he decided to make me a prom. We got dressed up and he put up decorations and cooked me a lovely dinner. No one had ever done something like this for me before. We danced a slow dance and I remember thinking how special I was to have found yet another great guy amongst the sea of evil I had intermittently experienced in my life.

Bryan and I spent most of our spare time together. This was a more mature romance than I'd had with my first boyfriend, John. We walked a lot, talked for hours. He listened and this was evident by his actions. There was a layer of me that he unraveled, and I was able to let him in. I was growing as a person, and he was a big part of the reason.

I don't know how I knew but I could tell that he would never hurt me. There were no expectations and I felt comfortable with him.

I knew he loved me. I'm not sure if he was *in* love with me but I know his feelings were deep and genuine. We had conversations about how he had never felt this way about anyone before and that I was special to him.

We only had a few short months prior to him leaving. But we made the most of the remaining time we had together.

I understood that there was a shelf life to what we had. I was never emotional during those days. I would never want anyone to see me cry. I had a wall of steel. So, when it came time to say goodbye, it was just that. I told him I would miss him. I kissed him long and hard and then he walked out of the door and then BAM!

My reaction to him leaving was so strong and unexpected. Tears streamed down my face. My chest was tight and heavy like someone was kneeling on me. I screamed. My body just gave way. I crashed against the wall and slid down to the ground with such force that I hurt myself. But the adrenalin was pumping so hard, and the grief just took over, so much so that I didn't realize until later.

I cried for hours. I'd think I was done, then I'd start again. I didn't move from that spot until later that evening. When I'd finally calmed down and pulled myself together, my head was fuzzy. I felt dazed and like I wasn't in my own body.

I decided to grab some food and watch a movie. Anything to take my mind off what I was feeling. I got battered sausage and chips with salt and vinegar. I deserved some goodies for afterwards. So, I picked up some chocolate bars and some diet coke to wash it down. I must have looked awful with my swollen red face. It was obvious that I had been crying, but no one said anything. I didn't care. When I wasn't crying, I was numb.

On the outside, I seemed like I knew a lot of people. I talked to everyone, but when it came to it, I only had one close friend in my life, and she was living her own life with her new boyfriend. I didn't want to bother her with my feelings, and I had no one else I could turn to.

I would spontaneously burst into tears. I tried so hard not to think about him. Yet, how could I not, when everything around me reminded me of him?

The portions from the chip shop were huge and filling. The aroma of the salt and vinegar was strong. I couldn't wait to dig in. I curled up on the sofa and watched tv as I ate. It tasted so good that I ate more than I should. I still ate the chocolate. Afterall, it's what you do when you break up with someone. Eat chocolate or ice cream, right? It's in all the movies.

After the realization that I was alone and I had no one to talk to, I started to sob uncontrollably again. My stomach was so full. As my belly bloated and the pain increased, all I could think of was that I needed the pain to stop. Still crying, I dragged my feet up the stairs to the bathroom. I immediately bent over the toilet, pushed two of my fingers down my throat until food came spewing out. The release felt good. The pressure was no longer there, and I was no longer in pain.

I know this seems like such an overkill. Believe me, I thought I was going crazy on this night. You have to understand that when I had someone in my life that I cared about, they ended up rejecting me. At least that was how I felt. Logically I knew that it wasn't as black and white as that, but my heart didn't see it that way. I was alone with only my emotions to keep me company.

This is when my life took a turn for the worse.

6

TWISTS AND TURNS

I needed to find a place closer to work. A girl I worked with told me about her friend. She had a room to let. I moved in right away. We never spent time together or tried to get to know each other. The conversation was strained, and there was an awkward tension whenever we would try too hard. I stayed in my bedroom most of the time.

I'd think about Bryan all day, every day. His absence in my life shook me to the core. I was consumed with replaying the last few moments we shared over and over. The more I got upset, the more I would turn to food for comfort. There was no intention of making myself vomit. Due to the junk, I'd eaten and being so emotional, I would end up with cramps and feeling horribly bloated, so I purged to feel better.

It was about once a week that I would be such an emotional wreck that I eventually felt ill and would end up releasing the discomfort. Then after a few weeks it became more often.

I lost a little weight and started to get compliments. Clients told me I was looking good. This stirred something in me, and I welcomed it. The more compliments I got, the better I felt. I could stop at any time, so I thought. I wasn't hurting anyone. I was in control.

A few weeks went by before I recognized that something had changed. I was purging when I didn't have pains in my stomach. It was usually after eating unhealthy food. It progressed to the point where I'd want to lose just a few more pounds, then I would tell myself that I was going to stop once I'd reached my goal. When I did, I didn't stop.

I didn't fully understand what I was doing, but I knew enough to know that it couldn't be healthy. I decided to make an appointment with the doctor.

I remember it like it was yesterday. I walked in wearing a baggy t-shirt and baggy work out bottoms. She asked me to sit down. I was nervous and didn't know what to expect. I clammed up. After a few moments of an awkward silence while she was reviewing my chart, I explained why I was there, and how I was feeling. She checked my weight and measured my height. With that she said I was in the normal range for my BMI and that there was no cause for concern.

The focus was on what I was consuming, and I explained that I was eating salads, soup, and other healthy meals between purges. She wasn't worried. She told me to come back if there was a drastic change in my weight. She said goodbye with a smile on her face.

I left thinking that if she wasn't worried, then I was ok.

My roller coaster of a life had so many twists and turns. I was unaware of the ride ahead. All too soon, the track reached the peak, and I was headed for the free fall, windswept and out of control.

I lost a little more weight, and I didn't want to put it back on. So, I purged after every high calorie meal.

There were days that I'd wake up so confident that I'd tell myself, this will be the day that I stop. I looked good and had no reason to continue. I would try so hard, but then would cave in when the guilt of what I had eaten set in.

The sticky tentacles of what I later learned was bulimia had well and truly had its grasp on me. I became obsessive and compulsive. The daily battle was intensifying with every day that passed.

My sister, Kelly, came to visit. She heard me one evening during a purge. Instead of talking to me about it she called my mum.

She asked me to take Kelly home. I did and when I was there, my mums' friend walked in and saw me and immediately burst into tears. It had been a while since they saw me, so it was a shock to see how I had changed.

Mum told me how worried she was and urged me to see a doctor. Her response when I told her what my doctor had said, was quite harsh. There really wasn't much said after that. Other than concern, she didn't know how, nor had the means to help me.

With something that started out so innocently, it quickly progressed into a need for control. It manifested so seam-lessly as it took a hold and became a dangerous game that fixated on food and weight. It was addictive. I'd get on the scales daily and if I put on weight, even a few ounces, I'd be so upset with myself and anxious that the readings would be higher next time.

I'd hoard food in my room and consume everything in private. I'd have a feeling of happiness while I was eating. It felt so good. Everything else in that moment didn't matter. The feeling was always temporary, though.

Although I wasn't aware at the time, I later learned that dopamine is released during overeating. This creates a sensation of pleasure and euphoria. This process allows us to continue the behaviour so that we feel good again, like posi-tive reinforcement. It helped me understand why I found it so hard to stop. By the time I learned this, it was too late.

My binges were always pizza, burgers, sweets, crisps, ice cream, and cake. I'd eat so much that my stomach would be so full and protruded that I'd look pregnant. I often worried that my stomach would burst.

My days became consumed with thoughts of food, types of food, ingredients, my caloric intake.

I'd struggle with the thought process of feeling like I was going to be good and the consequences if I weren't.

There was guilt immediately after eating and even more guilt knowing I'd purge. This turned to disgust at the thought of what I was going to do next.

Apprehension then took its turn. Will everything come up? On days that I felt more lightheaded, this quickly switched to, I should leave a little inside to keep me going.

This was my life.

It's hard to believe that with everything I was feeling, I was still a pro at putting on a façade. People saw the happy go lucky me. However, behind closed doors, without provocation, I was depressed and wanted to curl up into a ball and cry. I could die.

7

AT WAR WITH MYSELF

As the narrative of the new chapter in my life changed, I sank in the quicksand that bulimia had become. It continued to pull me down. My head was barely above the surface. I yearned to change my story, but without the courage to turn the page.

The me I once knew morphed before my very eyes. The irritable and deceitful person that reflected in the mirror was someone I no longer recognized.

*T*he urge took over. Waiting to get home to purge was no longer an option. I purged at work; people would complain about the smell.

Restaurants were a strategic battle against the comings and goings of the restroom. I would purge when it was loud and when no one was around, then stop as people came in. Making sure that I was never heard.

I would plan out my meal to ensure it was as easy to bring up as much as possible. I'd drink pints of water before and after each meal. This made it quick but often projectile and noisy.

People often commented and asked what I was doing to lose the weight. I'd tell them I was training for a half marathon. I lied all the time and had an answer for everything. I didn't even think twice about it. Like an addict desperate to hide the addiction.

Another level of anxiety would be added when I was staying at someone else's home. The last thing I wanted was for anyone to find out my secret. They wouldn't understand.

Everyone knew I loved bubble baths. So, this smoke screen was the perfect cover. The sound of the water running would drown out the sound of me vomiting.

The next level of cunning was born when I was faced with the overwhelming need to purge. I was in my room stuffing my face as usual, and my roommate was home watching tv in the living room. She would surely hear the sound of the vomit splashing against the toilet bowl. I needed an outlet that wouldn't give me away.

As the anxiety grew, I did the only thing of which I could think. I ran downstairs, grabbed a big black bin liner, and ran back to my room skipping every other step.

I put on some music. I knelt on the floor, gulping down water as I prepared myself mentally. I opened the bag as wide as I could and stared into it for a few seconds before I forced my fingers down my throat. I continued until I was dry heaving. My abdominal muscles hurt, and my throat was sore.

Surprised at how much was in the bag, I realize how much food and liquid I had consumed in one sitting. By this time, my stomach had stretched as it took more to fill me up than it once did.

The bag was heavy. I tied it securely and hid it in my room until I could find a time to take it out to the rubbish bin. Sometimes this had to be done in the middle of the night.

Once I knew that this was an option, it became a recurring thing.

Cravings would often take over and I'd knowingly eat something that would be harder to bring up like bread. It balls up and is lumpy as it passes your throat. The taste of the regurgitated food should have been enough to put me off, but I'd eat something to assist regurgitation like ice cream.

Purges were often planned. Especially the big ones. Leave work, purchase food, drink water, binge, drink more water and purge. This was the cycle.

More often than not, I'd become lightheaded immediately afterwards. It felt like my blood was leaving my body and I'd feel cold and start to sweat.

When this happened, I would be so adamant that I would stop. I needed to stop. I would wake up with the intention of not purging and having a healthy meal. I could quite often start the day on a good note or, my warped representation of what was good. I would skip breakfast, then would eat food, and wait. Then an overwhelming feeling of dread and anxiety would rise up in my body until I could no longer take it. Then the inevitable happened.

I was at war with myself.

Some days I would binge and purge 2-3 times a day. I'd be so weak that I'd have to eat some soup afterwards just to stop shaking and to get over the spaced-out feeling in my head.

Other days it would be once, and I would eat a healthy meal in between. On an exceptionally good day, I would eat healthy all day. There weren't too many days clumped together that were like that as I craved the high caloric foods.

The palpitations were a sign that my body was under duress. My heart felt like it was going to burst out of my chest, beating so fast and erratic, slowing down, then speeding back up, skipping a beat, sometimes catching my breath. This scared me.

What was I doing to myself?

As my body showed signs of wear, my personality followed suit. My self-esteem and self-worth plummeted.

I found myself doing things I could never have imagined. There were a few times when I was low on money, and I stole from the till at work. People would come into the gym and pay in cash. I took it. It wasn't for a rush, nor was it because I needed to pay bills. It was solely to fund my purge.

I am so ashamed of what I did and can't believe I turned into that person. If I needed money, all I had to do was ask my boss, he would have given it to me. That's the kind of guy he was. This has haunted me ever since.

Later, I did some research and found that it's quite common for those with eating disorders to steal. This doesn't make me feel any better. I don't want to feel better. I want to remember what I did and how low I was. It reminds me of how grateful I am to live the life I have now.

Whilst at a dinner party my roommate was hosting, I sat across from a guy that had ginger spikey hair. I remember smiling as it reminded me of a toilet brush. So, I secretly nicknamed him "bog brush." After dinner when everyone was drinking, he asked me to go upstairs where it was quiet, so we could chat. He seemed nice enough. Not my type, but we were just talking, and everyone was downstairs. So, no big deal.

He told me I was pretty and tried to kiss me. For the first time ever, I stood up for myself and turned away. I laughed a nervous laugh as he pulled me closer and tried again. He became very persistent and forceful and would not take no for an answer. I told him 'no', so many times. He didn't seem to care. He was laughing and acting like it was a joke. I was so sick and drained from fighting him off, I gave in. He laid me down and kissed me hard.

I was made more uncomfortable by the fact that we were in my roommate's room. I asked him to move in case she came up. He agreed. We were at the top of the stairs, all I had to do was walk down them. Why didn't I? I'll never understand the reason.

He grabbed my hand and led me to the spare room. He kissed me aggressively. It was rough, teeth clashing. I felt stuck and I knew what was about to happen. I didn't do anything. He lay me down and got on top of me.

Before I knew it, he was inside of me. I didn't want to. I didn't say no, again. There was no point. I let it happen. It's not rape, so what is it? What normal person allows this to happen?

That's not the sickest thing about this experience.

After that night, he kept calling me and asking my roommate to set us up. He hounded me and eventually I gave in again and I agreed to go to the movies. This was the start of the weirdest consensual *relationship* I could imagine. I hated him, he disgusted me. He repulsed me every time he touched me. I didn't find him attractive at all. I didn't like his personality. I didn't like him.

So, what was I doing?

I didn't tell anyone. If I couldn't understand why I could do this, then why would I ever think anyone one else could? Judgement was the last thing I needed.

I was emotionally disconnected from most people. I'd be so boisterous at work. It was fake. All I wanted to do was curl up on the sofa, watch TV and cry. I became withdrawn and reserved. There were only a few people that saw pieces of the real me. The me that was often hiding in the shadows.

Karli and I never really talked about the bulimia in detail. She didn't understand, and that was ok. It was glossed over. I don't even remember how it came up. She moved to a city just outside of London, so I didn't see her very often. But when we spoke on the phone, it always made me smile.

She was my rock in every other aspect of my life, but I was so ashamed and defensive that I kept that part of me at bay.

My friend Paul would visit when he could. I looked forward to seeing him. He grounded me. We had a true connection. His work had taken him to Phoenix, Arizona, but he would travel to England often during his trips to meet his customers.

Bryan and I were still in contact, and he asked if I'd like to visit him in the summer of 2001. I was twenty-one. I jumped at the chance. I knew we were just friends, of course. Even so, it was an amazing trip. His family was so generous opening their home and welcoming me with open arms. Their home was on a large piece of land that backed onto the woods. It was beautiful and relaxing. Just what I needed. We visited Chicago whilst I was there too. Navy pier was the highlight. The feeling I had in America was so different to how I felt in England. I felt lighter, happier, more myself.

I still purged. I did it when everyone was at work. I'd eat as healthy as I could in between. I didn't feel bad. In the clutches of bulimia, I never cared about anyone else except for me and what I was doing.

Back in England, feelings of panic would soon take hold.

I purged so often that I would lose my gag reflex. I'd be bent over the toilet so scared and panicked that I couldn't get the food up and it would become an ordeal. I'd shove my fingers so far down my throat that I'd get scars and red marks above my knuckles. I'd cry hysterically hitting myself. The verbal abuse I berated myself with was degrading. I even tried to use objects that were longer than my fingers and would damage my throat.

The act of violently making myself sick made me ill. I'd be on the floor so weak unable to move but still aware of what was happening.

Sometimes, the food would be so lumpy as it came up that it would get stuck in my throat. I couldn't breathe. I'd panic but was always able to dislodge it eventually.

Laxatives were taken by the handful. I'd have the shakes and cold sweats often, but the cramps were excruciating. It would trigger the palpitations. I'd be on the toilet so long. It just wouldn't stop. It was like a waterfall.

When it finally stopped, I would feel the effects for about 24 hours, sometimes longer. I was constantly on the toilet. The headaches and cramps were the worst. But the feeling of not really being in my right mind was right up there with it.

I wanted to stop, I told myself I was going to stop. But it had its grasp on me so tightly. Questions swirled around my mind like a tornado. Is this my life now? How would this end? Is there any point in going on?

8

FREEFALLING

During this difficult time, I had no emotional support from family or friends. People that may have had an inkling as to what was going on, looked the other way. I didn't think about the future. As I spiraled out of control and became more depressed, thoughts of giving up would creep into my mind. It's par for the course with bulimia.

It wasn't until later that I learned that bulimia was my survival mechanism, a coping strategy for dealing with underlying issues. The one thing I thought I could control. But in fact, it was bulimia that had control over me.

Christmas 2001 I got some news that Bryan was flying back for work. It was a short trip, but I was excited to catch up.

My employer was hosting a New Year Party. So, I invited him. It was a nice surprise to see Paul there. Bryan was so sweet. He told me it was ok to talk to Paul. The party overflowed into different rooms. So, I'd go and dance with Paul and then come back and spend some time with Bryan. He was leaving in a couple of days. He would always have a special place in my heart but we both knew that what we had was over.

A few days later, Paul surprised me by picking me up for lunch. He'd called ahead and cleared it with my boss, which was his best friend.

At lunch, Paul reached for my hand. It gave me goosebumps.

On the way back to work, he kissed me. I felt awkward and pushed him away. Only because I hadn't been kissed like that for a while. I didn't know what to do with it or know how I was supposed to feel.

Soon enough Paul was gone too. Back to America. But this time, he would call me nightly, and we talked for hours.

I wasn't in a good place. I couldn't trust myself, nor my instincts. My feelings were a tangled mess. I should have trusted others when they reached out in concern. I should have listened. Paul listened. He took the time to learn more about me. He asked questions that others were afraid to ask. And with that, we grew closer.

Time and distance were my friends. As I became more comfortable, I would disclose more about myself, opening up like a bleeding wound. I knew that it was just a matter of time before he came to his senses and realize I had too much baggage. But that time never came.

There was no judgment, only empathy. He listened and acknowledged my pain. He allowed me to feel my emotions. He told me to close my eyes and wrap my arms around him. He wanted me to imagine that his arms were around me. He told me to squeeze tight. He paused and told me he loved me.

This was a breakthrough. It was a monumental moment. We both fell in love.

I traveled to the USA to visit him. I was quite nervous about sex. Would Paul expect it? Would I be enough for him? Well, we did have sex and it was amazing.

He was so thoughtful and romantic. Our first official date was horseback riding at sunset to a steakhouse that was nestled amongst the mountains. Then he surprised me with a visit to Vegas. We had dinner in the Stratosphere where he told me he wanted to spend the rest of his life with me. He didn't propose, but it was more of a promise that it was on the horizon. I laughed, as it wasn't long ago that he told me he never wanted to get married. He said that I had changed his mind. I was the one.

He wanted me to go to England, pack and come back over as quickly as possible. When I was back in England, Paul had his friend John and his family over to visit. He told him everything about me. I wasn't sure how I felt about it. It was my personal struggle, my story to tell, but it turned out John already had his suspicions. He was the one that initiated the conversation and told Paul that people were complaining about the smell of vomit in the toilets.

Within weeks of being home, I found out I was pregnant. I was in shock. Paul was bound to freak out. I was on the pill, but of course with what I was doing, it wasn't the best method of birth control. We hadn't been together for that long. I called him and gave him an out. I had a history with cysts, irregular periods and now bulimia. This was not the best time for me to have a baby, but I couldn't help thinking, what if it were my only chance?

He did change his mind about marriage, but children? I needed him to understand that he was free to walk away. I wouldn't expect anything of him. Nor would I have any ill feelings toward him.

He was surprised. I could hear the fear in his voice. He held strong and told me not to worry. He would support me, and we would raise the baby together as a family. This solidified what kind of person I knew him to be. My heart warmed and I fell more in love.

I started to bleed. I panicked. Paul immediately left his friend and flew back to England to be by my side as the doctor gave us an update. Everything was good. We turned to each other and smiled as he squeezed my hand. In that moment I knew I really wanted the baby. He asked if I would move back with him right away where he could take care of me. My initial plan was to stay a while and tie up loose ends. He didn't like that idea.

We both stayed in a hotel for some privacy. We had dinner, a sip of champagne and he proposed to me. I was so happy. Luckily, he had already told me that he wanted to spend the rest of his life with me, or I could never have said yes, not just because of a baby anyway.

I moved to the US in March, right after my 22nd birthday. We got married in May. It was exciting in the beginning. An adventure. But then reality set in and things got difficult.

When I moved to the US, Paul was supportive, and he wasn't pushy. He let me know that I was loved and that he and our unborn child were great reasons to get better. He allowed me to find my own way to deal with everything so that I could get healthy again.

Moving to a new country was so much more stressful than I ever anticipated. I had no family or friends; I was emotionally unbalanced, and I was not able to work. I was independent in England and didn't realize how dependent I would be forced to become.

For me, life became a drudgery. I was unable to drive, and Paul was at work all day. The worst part was, I was hormonal and lonely. I had to rely on Paul and having someone support me was horrible. I hated asking for money, so I never really did anything. The struggle was emotional.

I felt so very much out of place. The terminology and food were different. No one got my humor. Even the way salespeople in shops would hover around me was annoying. It made me feel like I was about to steal something. I already had my own demons I carried with me. This made it worse.

Fashion styles were different. It was the desert, and I was used to lush green landscapes. Even buildings would cause me to be homesick. I was used to architecture that had history, cathedrals, castles, and the Monarchy.

The American accent was everywhere and was a constant reminder that I was an outsider. It's funny, now years later, I feel more out of place in England. America is my home, but not then.

Paul had no trouble with transitioning to the US. He loved it in Arizona. He had been here about six months prior to me, so he was established. Having me come over wasn't really a big deal to him. He went to work during the week, and we did fun stuff at the weekend. Aside from having me around, I don't think his life changed too much in the beginning.

He thought it would all fall into place when the baby was born. We were in the honeymoon phase of our relationship. It was me that felt the distance, but I tried to keep it to myself.

Anyway, all those things added to the bulimia. Pregnant and bulimic created a double-edged sword. I was living in a giant paradox. I was even more scared. I knew I was going to put weight on no matter what I did. This was something I couldn't control.

I'd be consumed about how it would affect me later. All I could think about was how much weight I was going to put on. Could I control it? Would it be hard to take off after the birth? I was nervous to tell Paul. Nevertheless, I was excited to have a human that would love me unconditionally.

Paul didn't fully understand what I was going through. He tried to learn about bulimia, but he couldn't find anything he felt could help me as a sufferer or something that would aid him as a supporter.

Initially he thought it was only a way to keep my weight down. At the time he didn't know the frequency of what I was doing or the health-related issues that it could cause. He assumed I could stop at any time, which caused much frustration. He thought it was a temporary thing. He had no idea that it was a mental health issue that had control of me.

As time passed, Paul struggled. We went to restaurants, and he'd watch me walk toward the toilets knowing what I was about to do. I could see the anxiety on his face. It killed him to stand by as I did this to myself.

Back then, he made it quite clear that it was a waste of time going to restaurants. He said it was a waste of money if I was going to throw it up anyway.

He told me it didn't change how he felt about me. He just wanted to understand so he could help me through it.

He'd try and make sure I had some healthy food that I'd feel comfortable keeping down. He tried to help me make better choices. Even so, I had bulimic thoughts all the time.

I started passing out when I was in my first trimester. While it can be common in early pregnancy, I had no idea that this would become more than just dehydration. It was a troubling and worrisome time. On many levels, there were things that contributed to the war with myself. You could easily say it became a decisive battle. I was putting my life and the life of my child on the line.

Sometimes I'd feel like I could eat a healthy meal and not purge. Paul often told me I had to for the sake of the baby. It was so hard. But if I ate healthy, and enough just to be satisfied and not get bloated, I could have good days. But, whenever I was unhealthy, this was a guaranteed purge day. The urge to binge eat was overwhelming. It was like an addiction. I felt so good when I binged, in that moment anyway.

I was torn between my illness and what I wanted for myself and battling against what was right for the safety of my baby. I also had to think about not disappointing Paul. It became about everyone else. As I got further along and could feel the baby kick, it became more real. It was motivation to do what was right. The struggle was real, but I had to try.

The last trimester was the hardest on my psyche. My emotions involving the pregnancy and body changes were erratic and draining. That's true to a certain extent in every pregnant woman, but bulimia compounded things and made me feel like I was caught in a vortex.

My doctors were concerned as I wasn't showing at all by 5 months and had only put on a few pounds by 6 months. That meant my baby was taking what nutrients he needed from me as I continued to lose weight. The baby measured small and needed to be monitored more closely throughout the pregnancy.

Supporting someone with bulimia had proven to be harder than Paul had expected. Once he realized being in a stable relationship and having a baby on the way wasn't enough to make me stop, his frustrations and lack of understanding would peer its angry head and we would argue. It would get vicious.

He was more aggressive during arguments. Then I would get defensive and reactive and scream and shout. We'd both say things we didn't mean.

The situation was perilous. My life and my baby's life were in danger and then my marriage. Everything I cared about was in jeopardy.

9

OUR NEW ARRIVAL AND AN OLD ENEMY

*P*aul and I were both excited about the prospects of having our baby, but we had no idea how to be parents. It was all new and the closer the due date came, the more anxiety we felt. Getting larger and feeling bloated much of the time, I really wanted to get into delivery. It was extremely important for me to push the baby into the world. I imagined enduring what every mother did and being rewarded with a beautiful baby laying across my chest, listening to my heartbeat from outside the womb for the very first time.

Our fights had become epic. I suppose it could be said Paul and I were passionate about how we felt. He wanted me to stop purging and I was doing all I could to comply. It wasn't easy. Paul went out of his way to be supportive, and it helped a great deal. He was my rock for sure.

The purging was better but then again, I was eating a lot less. I thought I was on the right track. Still, when I didn't eat enough, the baby didn't move or kick. It was frightening. Once I ate sufficiently, the baby became more active. The balancing act was overwhelming at times. I'm sure Paul was overwhelmed too.

With the delivery quickly approaching, we both had our concerns. Overall, we were in a good place. We wanted to be together, but it was hard. We went through a lot of difficulties. It was exhaustive. Yet, we remained affectionate and tried to work through things by talking them out.

There's only so much you can do as expectant parents waiting for the big day. You hope things will go well. When I finally started shopping for the baby, it was exciting. Looking at those tiny clothes that my baby would soon be wearing made me feel maternal and excited. I was motivated.

As a first-time mum with some health issues, I was worried. The closer the due date, the greater the anxiety. I'm sure Paul felt like I'd go into labor any minute. I was a week late, and I needed the baby to come. I was so uncomfortable, lightheaded all the time, I felt huge, I was anxious about the weight, and labor itself.

I had palpitations very often and it was a concern as to how bad it would get when I would have to push. I would try everything to trigger labor. Sex, spicy curry, running on the treadmill and raspberry tea as it was supposed to stimulate the uterus. Nothing worked.

I was induced with Pitocin, and still nothing happened. So, they sent me home. The next day at about 5am, I felt like I had wet myself. I didn't really know if he was pressing on my bladder, or if my water had broken. So, I called triage at the hospital.

They wanted me to go in just in case. I had tested positive for beta strep, so it was important that I had multiple rounds of antibiotics prior to delivery to ensure the safety of the baby. It turned out that my water had broken but I was not in labor. So, they had to try and induce me again.

It worked. The contractions came on strong. Aside from the vomiting that the pain caused and being tired and drained, labor was okay. I breathed through the pain until later that evening when I was just so tired, I ended up having an epidural. I never progressed and by 10:45pm I was told that I needed to have a C-section. I was in shock; I began to shake. I hadn't planned for that; I wanted a regular birth. I was scared, but I really wanted to push my baby into the world.

Paul was on edge. Excited and scared. He became anxious when I started shaking uncontrollably. My anxiety kicked in. I felt so out of control. I was a wreck and it made things worse. As they were about to cut me open, I moved. Luckily, Paul noticed, and they gave me an extra dose of medicine to make sure I was numb.

Connor finally arrived! I didn't get to hold him. Before I knew it, they whisked him away for testing. He was small but healthy! We were incredibly grateful. It was finally over!

I didn't react well to the anesthetic, especially having more of it.

I was a little zombified for a couple of days afterwards. I don't remember this; this is what Paul told me. I just remember feeling like I was having an outer body experience. Like I was experiencing everything from afar and that the emotions weren't lining up with what I was seeing.

Feeling so out of it when I met Connor, I felt weird. I thought I'd feel an overwhelming surge of love and adoration. I loved him, but there was a disconnect. I assumed it was because I didn't get to push him out. I was fixated on the fact that I needed to do this.

Initially in the hospital, it was like I was going through the motions of what a mum should do. It was nice to see him and hold him for a period, but I didn't mind when he was in the nursery or if someone else had him. I remember having odd thoughts. I questioned if he was my child. How would I have known if he was mistakenly switched? It was a while before I got to see him. This changed after a few days, when I looked at him and would see a mini-Paul staring back at me.

There was a time in hospital when I was alone with him, and he sounded like he was choking. I panicked and didn't think about the damage I could have done to myself, I just jumped out of bed and helped him. This protective instinct was a positive emotion amongst all the mixed feelings I kept inside.

He picked up nursing right away. This was lovely. I felt closer to him. Seeing Paul with Connor was heartwarming. Paul's face would light up. He was such a good, attentive father. It was delightful to see the two together.

I was able to bond with Connor better once we left the hospital. Still, something was missing, and it was disconcerting. Even Paul noticed it. For me, there was lots to deal with because the worries I had before delivery were now in the forefront of my mind.

I purged more when Connor was born, and once I healed from the surgery, I exercised Compulsively.

Loose skin, extra weight, stretch marks and all that goes with pregnancy, plagued me. I know this is superficial, but living with bulimia is hard enough, without adding uncontrollable factors to it. I knew pregnancy would make me lose control over my body. The anxiety about how I would look and feel after delivery truly bothered me.

My body had changed so dramatically that everything felt out of control. In a way, I was no longer me. Motherhood changes everything and not necessarily in a bad way. However, when you have bulimia and are dealing with those massive changes, it can wreak havoc on your emotions.

I was stressed and overwhelmed because my body was squishy. I purged and the weight came off very quickly, in a matter of weeks. That helped but we were still in the initial stages of adapting to a baby in the house.

I started feeling low, but I'd heard that some women got the baby blues shortly after giving birth. So, it didn't concern me. It got worse over time. I would feel better for periods and then I'd go downhill again. All of this had an impact on the bulimia.

I was nursing Connor and getting adjusted to that. It did help with the bonding but there was this persistent feeling that things weren't right. I was depressed and often detached. That's not how things are supposed to be. I had strong regrets that dug a pit inside me: That I didn't try hard enough to protect my baby. That I lied to Paul often and told him I hadn't purged when I had. That I kept how I was feeling to myself most of the time as I was scared to disappoint Paul. I felt like a failure.

I should have reached out for professional help, to talk to someone about it and work though my feelings. It was Paul that noticed that something was wrong. I just felt like I wasn't one of those mothers that doted on their kids or wanted to be with them 24/7. I was different, I just didn't know how. I didn't think anything was wrong. I just thought I was more emotional.

Paul was always helpful. He did the laundry, cleaned, ironed and was amazing with Connor. The only thing we butt heads on in the beginning was that he thought I should be the only one to get up in the night since he had work. I didn't agree. This caused conflict.

We talked through it, and he understood that it was important to my mental health that I needed to get more sleep. It was his idea to take turns to get up for him in the evening. This helped a lot. I pumped milk for his nights, and it worked out.

I was purging more during this time. I was torn as I needed to eat to be able to produce milk, but I quickly realized that my milk was not producing like it should. Connor was still small, and the pediatrician told us that he was low on the percentile scale and should put more weight on.

Every day was long, and I felt inadequate. All I did was stay at home with a baby. I kept thinking; my life was meant to be more than this. I didn't really feel joy. I was unable to work due to my visa status. I had a couple of friends but to them, I was happy, and life couldn't be better.

Paul and I began to argue again, so often and so hard that there would be holes in the walls. We were both adjusting to our new life, but it was more than that.

He would get so hot headed and let his frustration out by hitting the wall. I'd be defensive and would react with so much anger I'd do the same. I can't remember the number of times I said the words, "I want a divorce," or "I can't take it anymore."

We can laugh at this story now. Back when things started getting better for us, our friendly pest control guy came over to our new home and asked, "So, you and Paul doing better?" When I questioned why he thought that, he laughed and responded with "There are no holes in the walls." It was pretty funny.

There were other things that weren't funny at all. I felt like a bad Mum, like I didn't deserve to have Connor. I think the more I thought like this, the more distant I became. I was happy just to watch Paul be with him. It was such a chore to do things for him for extended periods of time and this made me hate myself.

It was a dark time for Paul. My bulimia was problematic, and I was passing out. Not only did Paul have our newborn child, now he had my mood to deal with. He tried hard to make me feel better by doing things together but I'm sure he was so tired that he just wanted it to change. He was worried. I knew I needed help, but I didn't go to a doctor. I'm not sure why.

I didn't know at the time, but women that battle with bulimia, are at greater risk for postpartum depression. Many women have postpartum blues following delivery that can last for about 2 weeks. I learned later that, experiencing symptoms longer than this, could manifest into something more serious.

Feeling hollow inside was yet another sign that I may have been suffering from postpartum depression. As I mentioned, I did have that disconnect immediately. It did let up for a while, but then it always came back.

I wish I weren't so defensive and understood that Paul was coming from a place of concern. He didn't intentionally hurt my feelings or want to make me feel bad. He was worried.

I'm not sure if it's because I didn't do anything, that it manifested into regular depression. Or if it was the Bulimia, or a mixture of everything.

As Connor grew, other incidents triggered strong reactions in me. He would kiss me on the lips. This felt inappropriate. It happened a lot and was disturbing to me. Even when he got older and nestled his head in my chest, it felt wrong. In hindsight, it brought back to the surface the abuse I experienced when I was young.

During the pregnancy and Connor's early years, Paul and I would argue constantly. We'd have good days and bad days. I felt like I wanted to leave a lot. I just wanted to run away from the feelings. But we would ask each other if we wanted to make it work. We did. The love was there but I often wondered if that was enough.

It wasn't until Connor was about five that Paul gave me an ultimatum. I get help for the depression, or he would walk away. The lack of emotion, lack of involvement in Connor's life and worrying about the bulimia was just too much. He had dealt with it all for so long and I wasn't doing anything to get better. He couldn't see an end in sight.

Paul wanted us to work and to be a happy family, but he had to know that I was serious about working on myself and the bulimia. Not just for him and Connor, but for myself.

The day I walked into the Doctor's office took me back to the time when I first reached out for help. The fork in my life that could have sent me on a different path if only my doctor was educated on eating disorders.

I sat with my feet tucked under my bottom as I cried and told my story. The doctor listened and allowed me to say what I needed to without interruption. He welcomed the silences that came so that I could digest everything before asking open ended questions when he felt I was ready. I felt a glimmer of hope.

That day I started an anti-depressant medication and within a month or so I felt lighter and not as emotionally burdened.

Paul and I had a heart to heart. He made me think about how the future would look if I continued down the same destructive path and how it could look without the bulimia. We talked about the life I wanted and made me decide if I wanted him in it.

We were all in. I chose him, our family. With a promise to strive for a healthy future, we started the long winding bumpy road to recovery.

10

LIKE SUDDEN DEATH

*P*aul asked me what he could do to help me. What I needed from him, and we devised a plan together which was important. No dictation of what he thought I needed.

He agreed to do some research as I told him that I felt he didn't understand what I was going through and that prevented me from baring my soul to him, as I felt his anguish and disappointment.

I needed him to understand the fundamentals of my eating disorder. He needed to hear from a professional's perspective on what can cause bulimia, and how the sequence of binging and purging can be triggered in response to stress, anxiety, and depression.

It's so crucial to have a strong support system. One that is educated and will positively reinforce all the small steps that are made towards recovery, instead of being made to feel guilty and a failure for the times that we slip up. This can be a trigger and send anyone struggling with bulimia into a downward spiral.

It's possible that all those small changes could one day add up and over time the good will outweigh the bad.

Paul eagerly learned and absorbed all that he could find. It was easier this time around. There was more information available.

The more he researched and realized the harm I was inflicting upon myself, the more he was scared. The pieces of the jigsaw puzzle were slowly starting to fit in place as he uncovered other characteristics of bulimia other than self-induced vomiting. Prolonged fasting, abuse of laxatives and diuretics, and obsessive exercise.

Knowing that I'd be battling with this for life and the thought that I could die at an early age from heart failure, scared him most. Bulimia didn't develop overnight. We both knew that my recovery would not happen overnight either.

I continued to struggle but with Paul's love, support, and continued efforts, my trust grew. I no longer needed to defend myself or explain why I couldn't just "keep it down."

Our 'check in' conversations became more frequent, and I found myself digging deeper into the past and divulging things that had been locked away.

There were often tears, but telling my secret was like therapy.

Once the pain was unleashed, I allowed myself to think about the cause of it. I acknowledged it and gave it the time it deserved. Then I made a conscious decision to put it aside and vowed it would no longer control me.

Paul reassured me that he was here, he loved me, and no one was going to hurt me again. This was when he could link the information that he'd learned with my story.

With this new understanding, I felt the empathy flooding back into him. That look of disappointment faded away and was replaced with unconditional support and an overflow of love that beamed down on me again.

He acted like a sponsor. If I felt the urge to binge, he'd want me to talk to him about what I was feeling and asked if I'd recognize what may have brought it on. He'd take the time to talk through it and would take my mind off that moment and offer to go for a walk or to do something fun.

This often worked prior to binging. Not all the time, but it did help. I also struggled on days where I had no triggers, I just craved the binge.

It was so hard. It caused anxiety to have food inside of me. It was my goal to keep food down as long as possible before purging. That way I would absorb more nutrients. Then gradually, I would have longer periods in between purges. I yearned for the day to come when my life wasn't consumed and fixated with food.

I'd have setbacks all the time. After a purge, I'd feel disappointed in myself. Feeling down, I would tell Paul and surprisingly he always reacted with love. He'd tell me that he was proud of how far I'd come. He'd say that setbacks are to be expected during recovery and I just had to get back up from this and fight another day. He'd hug me and tell me he loved me.

He'd kiss me on the forehead and rest his chin on the top of my head as he hugged tighter. Even today, whenever Paul can sense that I'm having a stressful day or that I have something on my mind, he'll stop what he's doing and kiss me on the forehead. This always makes me smile. It reassures me that we are in tune, that he is aware of my emotions, and he is here for me.

He'd make healthy meals and make sure to portion control, so I was less likely to get bloated and feel the need to purge.

He kept me occupied by filling weekends with fun activities to look forward to.

He told me I was beautiful all the time. He was present in my life and active on my road to recovery.

When I was younger, I'd keep a diary and would write poems to express my feelings. Paul encouraged me to write about my story as a release and a way to heal. I wanted to, but I was never ready.

Years had passed and I was still fighting the battle with bulimia.

I found myself going a week without purging, then two. Every time I relapsed, I just started again. It was emotional but over time I had more good days in a row.

Although I was on my way to achieving a victory in the war with bulimia, there were many times where the battle got the best of me.

I was periodically blacking out and one day when I was hospitalized, I was sent for some tests. One of them was a tilt table test. This is where you are strapped to a table, and your body position is adjusted from horizontal to vertical. The test can tell your doctor if faulty brain signals are causing low blood pressure which causes the fainting. This is when I was diagnosed with Vasovagal Syncope.

It's an overaction to the vagus nerve and can cause a sudden drop in your heart rate and blood pressure. It happens when the blood vessels open too wide, or the heartbeat slows too much, causing a temporary lack of blood flow to the brain.

When I pass out, my heart rate is so low Paul can barely feel my pulse. It feels like sudden death, except that you wake up.

The scariest time was when I woke to find him hovering over me about to do CPR. He couldn't feel my pulse at all, and I wasn't waking up as quickly as I usually did. I can't imagine what was going through his mind.

It can be triggered when I exert myself, get stressed out, if I get up too quickly, get emotional and for no reason at all. I'm under the care of a cardiologist and it was recommended I put on weight to reduce the frequency of the Vasovagal Syncope. This was a hard pill to swallow.

Something I learned along the way was that patients with bulimia should be monitored for cardiovascular complications such as this. If you're reading this and you relate to anything I've mentioned, I urge you to seek medical advice. It's essential to confide in your doctor. Explain what you've been struggling with and any symptoms you may be experiencing. It's important to be honest.

Fainting can indicate other serious things and it's best to determine the actual cause of the fainting. We know that mortality is doubled for those who have Vasovagal Syncope.

Every year there are 500,000 new patients. Yet, even more people may suffer from the disorder. It is estimated that 50% of people don't seek care until after their second incident.

If you notice the early warning signs of fainting, you may be able to circumvent a black out. If you start to feel warm, or cold and clammy, it's recommended to sit down and put your head between your knees and grunt or cough. Lying down with your legs in the air is best but it may not always be possible in public.

Paul has had a great deal to manage with my fainting. No doubt he's constantly worried if I'll wake up – this time. The stress must be tremendous. I'm glad he's been there for me. It's made a huge difference. He has made a huge difference.

11

LIFE 2.0

There are two types of people in the world. Those that complain about negative things that happen in life, projecting that energy into the world, thus attracting more of that same energy back into their life. They get stuck in this never-ending cycle. They are often unhappy and lack a fulfilled life. These people bypass the outreached hand of chances that are put in their path as they are oblivious to anything outside their bubble and quite often are unable to see the forest for the trees.

Then there are those that appreciate what they do have, are grateful for the things they receive and are aware of their surroundings and see opportunities where others don't, and act on them.

I was living in limbo. The space in between. I never complained about anything I experienced or was going through, but I was never profoundly grateful for what I had or appreciated the life that was available to me. I allowed people to drain my energy and suck the life-force I had worked so hard to build up.

In my 30's I recognized that I had to put in more work. I needed to make some additional adjustments if I were to live a life that would make me smile every day.

I started immediately and the world around me evolved.

The trees seemed greener, the sun brighter and the people nicer. Things slowly started changing until one day, I noticed I felt different. Warmer. Softer. More joyful. Fulfilled. At peace. I was finally learning to live a life that I dreamed of. A life that I deserved.

The journey to become a better me was initiated by cutting off the energy vampires. My emotional energy belonged to me. And only me.

I needed to increase my positive energy and rebuild the relationship with my family.

Paul and I implemented a monthly date night that was not focused on food. We took turns in surprising the other with a fun activity. Time and effort went into planning something that the other was sure to like. We both appreciated this. We went sky diving, horse riding, and shooting at the range. We enjoyed picnics at the lake and staycations in local hotels so that we could spend quality time together, even if it were just around the pool talking. This was a big step in rebuilding the foundation of our relationship that I very nearly destroyed.

Family time was more abundant with fun activities, games nights and mini vacations. We laughed more and enjoyed each other's company more than ever.

The more I freely gave and took time to be present in each moment, the more I got back in return. The better I felt emotionally, the more it showed in the decisions I made. It paved a new path for me to follow. A path I was finally ready to take.

After more than 15 years of no contact with my dad, I learned that he had cancer and had reconnected with my mum. Divorced for a second time he found himself going through his own battle, alone. Mum hated to see him vulnerable and uncomfortable. She supported him in any way that she could. She was there for him as he suffered through his treatments, helped him with housekeeping and was there for him emotionally when needed. This was not out of obligation, but out of compassion. Over time their feelings grew into more and the spark that was once there, began to ignite again.

This kicked up a lot of emotions for me, but for my mum's sake I never confronted my dad.

I could have chosen to continue to think of my dad with such disdain as I had for years. Remembering how he broke my heart and my spirit as a child. Or I could take this opportunity for what it was. A chance to reconnect.

My mum spoke to my dad at length about what it was like for me growing up without him. How his decisions impacted me with such force that it was like a tornado tearing through a city and leaving the remains scattered in pieces.

Over the years my dad had changed. His lifestyle, his personality and demeaner was now something that my mum recognized from back in the day. This was the man she was once in love with, and something told me that he could be again.

My dad tried. First with texts and sometimes a call. They were superficial conversations and were often strained, but he was trying. I didn't know him, and he didn't know what to say to me, so it was hard.

I made the decision to take control of the emotions that talking to my dad evoked. I read The Language of Letting Go by Melody Beattie. This book promotes taking responsibility of our own self-care. She reminds us to remember that each day is an opportunity for growth and renewal. Her daily meditations focus on self-esteem, acceptance and letting go. The best thing about this book is that it can be applied to anything you want to let go of. Emotional burdens, guilt, loss of a loved one, a feeling of wrongdoing, infidelity and so on.

As an extension of this, I visited a hypnotherapist. She triggered my pain and forced me to imagine it in a physical form, as a ball of light. I moved the pain gradually from my toes, feeling it building as it passed my hips. It was the strongest as it reached my heart. I was sobbing uncontrollably, but it was something I had to do.

As it made its way through my arms, I reached out in front of me and released the ball of light that enveloped my pain, my anguish and resentment and, I let it go. It doesn't matter if you believe in hypnotism or not. The act of going through this exercise is so impactful that I use this whenever I feel anxious or nervous about something.

I didn't know that it had worked until I had watched a movie about the turbulent relation between a father and his daughter and realized it didn't make me cry like it had so many times before.

My dad and I will never be close, but I can honestly say that the space that used to house the animosity I felt toward him, is now filled with love. I'm happy to have him in my life.

With an open heart and a positive mindset, I took every day as it came. Whenever I had a bad thought or felt down, I would bring my attention back to all the good I had in my life. I was making progress and my life kept getting better.

It was through serendipity that I found a career that I loved, in the mortgage industry. I especially enjoyed, and still do enjoy, working with first time homebuyers as the excitement they have fuels my feel-good tank. This was a huge boost to my self-esteem. I started contributing to the household in a meaningful way. My sense of self-worth was stronger, and I felt more in control of my life than ever before.

I desperately wanted to give back. It felt good. Soon enough I would find myself in a situation where I could do just that.

I made an appointment to have my hair colored. My stylist was in her 20's and the energy around her was full of sadness. I recognized myself in her demeanor and was drawn to her for some reason. As we talked, I found out why. She was comfortable opening up to me and the floodgates opened. She was homeless and had no family support. Her background was so eerily similar to mine, that my heart ached for her. She started drinking to self-medicate and felt like her life was spiraling out of control.

She was jumping from job to job as she couldn't hold anything down. Her dream job was teaching in a beauty school but felt like it was an unobtainable dream. We exchanged numbers and I asked her to call me so we could get together after her shift.

I called Paul and expressed my concern. I had an overwhelming urge to help her, and I needed Paul to be ok with it. I couldn't bear to know that someone was hurting and couldn't see a way out ahead. I know firsthand where that can lead.

I don't know why I was so surprised by his response. But it showed how much he loved me and supported me. Knowing how much I yearned to help people, he told me to call her right away and invite her to live with us. We had a guest room that wasn't being used. The least we could do was offer it. She started to cry and said yes. She could stay as long as she needed. We didn't expect anything in return. We wanted her to rely on us for support so that she could get back on her feet.

She did everything she set out to do and became a manager and teacher at a beauty school and got her own apartment.

I feel selfish knowing how much this made me feel good.

I made more progress. Before I knew it, a month had passed without purging. When I relapsed, I wouldn't get too down, I'd concentrate on what I'd accomplished. But I had to be incredibly careful that I didn't think too much about the feeling of release it gave me, as it would be too easy to go down that slippery slope. It's addictive.

Even though I went longer without purges, I was still strict with my food and everyday was hard work. I was still consumed with thoughts of food and how my body would change if I didn't work out as hard.

When I got back from Spain my body type changed and became one that bulked easily around my thighs. So many fitness experts out there tell you that it takes a lot for this to happen but, try telling that to all the woman I have spoken to that feel the same way.

Early in my recovery it was extremely hard not to purge knowing I'd put on weight and was made even more difficult knowing that I'd be unhappy with the way I looked.

At the height of the Bulimia, I was laser focused on working out hard, heavy, fast, and burning as many calories as possible. I was exercising excessively at a high intensity, and it wasn't doing me any favors.

I went back to the fundamentals I learned when I worked in the fitness industry and researched fun new exercises that resulted in a leaner look. It wasn't anything I didn't already know, but now I was willing to slow down and continue at a healthy pace.

I implemented my new workout routine, and I couldn't be happier. I feel great about myself and knowing that I will never bulk up with my workouts helps me stay on track. Not only on a physical level but psychologically too.

I stay away from anything that has the potential to build too much muscle around my thighs, such as cycling, ellipticals, cross-trainers and stepping machines. This included inclines when I'm on the treadmill too. Squats, lunges, deadlifts, and heavy lifting are also a thing of the past.

If you'd like to see what could possibly be left after I had eliminated all of this, or you feel like it's something that could benefit you or a loved one, then check out the workout regimen on the downloadable pdf I've put together to get you started. https://linktr.ee/WarWithMyself

Meditation was recommended to kick start my day stress free. I learned that being mindful can give you a sense of calm, peace and balance that can benefit your overall well-being. It can alleviate stress, help with anxiety, help you sleep better, focus your attention and so much more...

It made such a positive impact on my day that I continued, and now I meditate daily. Taking the time for myself to do breathing exercises and start the day on a positive note, paves the way for a better day.

I start by finding somewhere calm and quiet and play some relaxing music or spa sounds. Sitting with my legs loosely crossed and my hands on my knees with my eyes closed, I take slow deep breaths. In through my nose as deeply as I can and out through my mouth as long as I can.

Keeping my mind clear and focused was hard in the beginning. I had to keep bringing my attention back to my breathing. Feeling my breath as I breathed in and breathed out.

Where was this all my life? I'd heard about the benefits for years, but until I experienced the calming effects for myself, I could never have understood. This tool alone helps bring balance to a moment where you need clarity, calm, if you need to reset your day or to unwind at the end of a stressful day. Whatever the reason, you'll be sure to take something away from it. Try my guided meditation to relaxation and letting go https://linktr.ee/WarWithMyself

That first day I made myself vomit; I had no idea that 20 years later I'd still be fighting to stay healthy. But the more control I took over my feelings and the harder I worked on myself by researching and implementing new tools and techniques to aid in my recovery, the happier I became. My marriage was stronger than it had ever been. I was winning more battles and I had hope that the war would soon be won.

Journaling was a way I continued to work through my feelings. Writing the highlights of my day whilst smiling, and feeling the emotion was a good boost. The low points were added, but instead of leaving it there, I would add how I overcame them. If there was anything unresolved, I would bullet point a plan of action to accomplish what was needed to settle my mind.

When I had a bad day, I would write down all the negative feelings. I'd acknowledge the emotion it triggered and then I would cross them out and replace them with something positive I wanted to feel in that moment. I'd highlight those words, close my eyes, and think about them for a few minutes. This always brought me back to a better emotional state.

The more I used all that I had learned, the more I realized why I hadn't been successful in my recovery until now.

My 'ah ha' moment was when I heard something on the radio about nourishing your mind, body, and soul. This was it. The key to it all. The missing elements.

It isn't enough to eat healthy and hope that nothing triggers a purge. Staying strong emotionally and physically through working out is important, but also, isn't enough.

Dealing with your emotions from past traumas is a crucial part of the healing process, but on its own, it isn't enough.

Taking time to yourself to reflect and relax, giving back and being grateful for what you have, all have healing properties, but unfortunately, it just isn't enough.

Tears began to form when I grasped what this meant. I needed mind, body, *and* spiritual fulfilment. I needed to embrace and feed it all. This was the prescription for my happy, healthy, and fulfilled life.

So, I continued my journey with outstretched arms as I went longer and longer without the need to purge.

Daily Affirmations became a mainstay: To motivate, inspire and be a daily reminder that I can live a positive lifestyle. I'd find positive things I wanted to believe in, and I'd say them aloud whilst looking in the mirror.

- I am beautiful
- I am strong
- I am a survivor

- I don't need my eating disorder to be good enough
- Today I will abandon my destructive behavior
- Today I will use behaviors that are good for me

The personality that everyone sees, is the true me.

No more hiding, no more feeling less than.

The metamorphosis was enlightening. I believed in myself. I was full of joy. Every aspect of my life had improved. This is when I started to meet some amazing friends one by one. They just so happened to be from the UK. We named ourselves the Brit Chicks. An uplifting group of girls that connected over a shared history. Girls that rally around one another when needed. Who laugh together to lift our spirits, pick each other up when we fall and of course have some good old fun.

From here my recovery seemed to be on warp speed. With all the positive changes in my life, I made sure to give back.

My daily gratitude is something that makes me smile. On my drive to work, I look out at the mountains and say aloud what I am thankful for. Good things that had happened the day before, my fur babies, another day without purging, my amazing family. Anything for which I am truly thankful. It's important to give back, even if all you have to give, is what you're thankful for.

The more I give the better I feel, the better I feel, the healthier I stay, and more good things come into my life. So, why wouldn't I continue?

Paying it forward and doing a good deed is a staple in my life now. Doing little things that I know will make people feel good fuels my energy. Paying for someone's coffee, giving a compliment, letting someone go ahead in line. It doesn't have to be big or expensive, just thoughtful. The more you give back the more it makes you feel good. Creating these small emotional changes can build into something bigger. Over time it could make a positive impact on your emotional wellbeing.

PRESCRIPTION FOR VICTORY

When our mothers first hold us just after we're born, do they wonder what roads we will travel? As children, we don't know the journeys we will take in real life, but we pretend to be all sorts of things as we find our way down the road.

Along the way, sometimes horrible things happen to children, things that change their course in life and even the way they think about things and how they view people. Some children no longer know how to view themselves. They look in the mirror not liking what they see.

*T*he sordid realities being too painful are stuffed deep down inside, compartmentalized, and sealed away. Yet, those memories ever fresh, ever painful find ways of getting out. They must be dealt with before they eat away at our very existence. I know.

Parents often prefer their children to be silent, to be seen and not heard. That too, can cause frightful repercussions. In my case, the burden of the incidents that happened in my life got too heavy to carry. So, my mind, and my emotions seemed to turn on me.

Enduring repeated traumas without understanding what was really happening seared the events in my mind. Not understanding and not being rescued can lead to many things. In my case, it led to bulimia. The disease set me on a path, like a gerbil on an exercise wheel. Around and around I would go, never getting anywhere.

When I stopped running, I started eating, binging, and then purging. The dopamine fix eased the pain and the memories briefly. The addiction was so strong that I had to stay on that wheel, running with all my might, then binging, and purging.

Connections were formed in my brain by the chemicals released making lasting impressions. My behavior was fixed on a dangerous pattern that could have killed me. My heart, longing to be free, to love and be loved, could stop at any moment.

Palpitations and black outs ruled the day. Anxiety and fear ruled the night. I was destroying myself from within. The enemies, the people who oppressed and abused me were ever present, but I became my own worst enemy. The weapon I used on myself was powerful. I never ran out of ammunition. Systematically, I set out to destroy the child and then the adult who didn't comprehend the damage done by interlopers. I couldn't comprehend the enemy within.

With help and with love, I began to see that there was hope for me. I fell many times but with encouragement, support and love I was able to get back on my feet to try again.

Our minds and lives are fragile. Our interactions and relationships with others are even more fragile. Daring to try, daring to find love, daring to *be* loved, my detour was mapped out. The journey on the road from nowhere to somewhere began. The highs and the lows of love at times were no threat to the dopamine dump into my system, but with time love conquered all.

Paul was my lifeline, my rock, and my joy. Our son gave me purpose to think about getting better. The struggle will always be there, but my family buoys me, strengthens and guides me to shore when I drift into old habits.

An armistice was declared, and fighting stopped. Occasionally, there would be skirmishes followed by a cease fire that lasted for a while. The skirmishes diminished as I found myself, as I forgave myself. Life goes on if you let it and it can be beautiful.

Now, I have a good relationship with my family and still have a relationship with my dad. Paul and I are stronger. We grew together and closer to one another. We adopted a little girl who is fighting her own war, and although it has been a struggle, that journey has been worth it. My son has gone off to university and I couldn't be prouder. They all survived the strafing runs associated with bulimia. They loved me despite the conflicts.

I'm still working successfully in the mortgage industry and found a wonderful team to grow with and look forward to going to work each day.

Happy and healthy, food does not have a hold over me now. I can enjoy food but overall, I eat more healthily. I am still aware of my emotional state and how it can affect my mood. I still have to be conscious about my thoughts to ensure the weakness that underlies my psyche does not crack it wide open.

I've retrained my brain. Just like training your body, it's hard work, but the end result is worth it. I am happier with my body now than I have ever been and don't mind my imperfections.

I changed the focus I used to have behind the closed doors of the bathroom. What once was a place to cover the sounds of vomiting, now mimics a relaxing scene from a movie. I made new memories. Relaxing in a bubble bath, surrounded by candles listening to calming music. This is my time to reflect and feel any emotion I need to, to acknowledge them and let them go.

I give my emotions the time that's needed, releasing the built-up tension. I allow myself to cry. For a reason, for no reason at all. Just another release. I come out of the bathroom feeling better. Like I had a therapy session.

I'm doing what my husband suggested and am writing down my feelings. In the process it turned into a story that I realized could help people. You have your own story about how you began your journey. Honor the process and honor yourself. Love yourself. If you can love yourself as you should, destructive behavior diminishes. Once you love yourself, you're able to love someone else and you allow them to love you.

You can win your war with yourself. You will find the right prescription that will lead to peace. Merely existing in life is not what we're born to do. Being chained to our emotions and to the destructive inner processes is no way to live. Life is worth it. You are worth it.

LETTER TO THE SUFFERER

FROM ME TO YOU...

*W*hether you know it or not, by reading my story you have taken a step towards understanding your illness and making a conscious decision to improve your health.

My hope is that you read something that resonates with you and encourages you to step back and assess your own situation. Maybe it's helping you realize that your eating disorder is attached to an emotion which is stemmed from a particular life event. Or showing you that others do shameful things throughout their illness too. You are not alone. There are many like us that have struggled and are continuing to struggle along the same path. But it's important to highlight how much we can learn from those that have come before us. And in my case, through sharing my own experience, I want to help those that follow. That includes you.

It's important for you to know that I firmly believe that if I had talked to a professional, and have implemented all that I have, I would have likely gotten though my years of recovery more quickly. The reason I didn't, was because of my lack of trust based off one uneducated doctor all those years ago.

It took a lot of trial and error trying to do it on my own. It only slowed my recovery. It almost destroyed my marriage. I felt like a shadow of my former self, and I was miserable for 20 years of my life.

Healing physically, emotionally, and psychologically are the key factors to obtaining a balanced and healthy life after enduring our darkest time. I do believe this. I'm not saying that if you follow the same steps as I did during my recovery, that you're going to be better immediately. It takes hard work and time. But what I can say is that during my research on treatment centres and therapists that treat patients with eating disorders, their treatment plans are well rounded and include most of what I implemented. There is something in it. Trust me.

If there's even a little part of you that is tired of continuing down this destructive path, day in and day out, then I urge you to start your own journey, now!

There is hope and as you can see, there are steps you can take to aid in your recovery.

Start the healing process from any trauma you've experienced and be open to forgiveness. It will help you move on.

If you don't, it can manifest into anxiety and depression. You may feel like you're ok, that you're handling it, but if you look closely to your personality traits, you may see that you have changed.

Are you more reactive, aggressive? Your trauma may be the contributory factor.

I know it's hard but confront your guilt. Stand head on with your anger and fight back against all your frustrations.

The feeling of shame, self-disgust, lack of self-esteem and self-worth is a shared feeling amongst sufferers. It's ok to acknowledge that you feel this way and why, but you don't need to stay in this space.

Repetition takes power away from your story. So, start by opening up to someone you trust and continue to talk about it. It works.

Be vulnerable, acknowledge the feelings, own it, and let it go.

If you'd like to start your journey by confiding in me, I'm here to listen. As someone that has walked in your shoes.

LETTER TO THE SUPPORTER

WORDS OF ENCOURAGEMENT

*F*irst, I want to say, I hear you. I understand that you are in unknown territories. Not knowing how to help your loved one can be heart wrenching, scary and frustrating. Your feelings are valid.

No matter how many times you may have been told, *it's not about you,* you are a big part of the recovery process. So don't give up.

Once you are past the initial shock of discovery, then there are things you can do to help.

I'm not sure if you've realized, but the more you push, the more it could have an adverse reaction. Be mindful that what you say and do can be a trigger.

Educate yourself so you understand the illness and can recognize the cyclical behavior it possesses. Only then, will you truly have the foundation a supporter needs.

Whether you know it or not, your loved one has likely experienced something that made them feel out of control. They may not yet understand this themselves, so coming hard and heavy with 'Why are you doing this to yourself?' may not be reciprocated with an answer.

And telling them to "just eat" will alienate you.

You could end up starting an argument, or they could retreat in silence. I'm not sure which one is worse. This will likely end with them feeling emotionally beaten and distressed. They will find themselves again, in a situation where they feel worse about themselves and could end up binging to feel better and ultimately doing the very thing you wish them to stop... purging.

You may find it difficult to comprehend but your loved one finds security in their illness.

People find it hard talking about the pain they carry. Even though it may be heavy on their heart, they can hide it very well.

From experience, we always keep secrets that we think we have to hide. We are always on overdrive, so we don't have to feel the pain. Although your loved one might initially try to push you away, they still need to know that they are not alone.

Express your eagerness to help because you love them.

Be open about what you've learned. Be compassionate and show that you are interested in understanding what they are going through.

Don't be scared to ask what you can do to help.

Start your conversations when you are out on a walk so it reduces the anxiety that will surely arise. Don't be confrontational.

Don't push. Explain that you wish to have more understanding and that you are there for them. The silent questions you have, may go unanswered for a while. Your loved one, may not feel safe enough to talk in the beginning, but over time, they may surprise you.

Periodically, ask them if they are ready to talk to a professional. But if they refuse, and are more comfortable talking to you, then help them to acknowledge any emotions that they are feeling and what may have triggered them.

Underlying issues are about emotional suffering and pain, not food.

So, if your loved one can talk openly about the pain then it could be a step toward recovery.

They need to accept that they are no longer in control. They need to understand the reason their eating disorder manifested, take responsibility for where they are right now and have a plan of action for future goals.

Show positive reinforcement with every achievement. They may not show this appreciation, but it goes a long way.

Passing judgement, fault or blame is a sure way to put distance between you. So, don't make them feel guilty for a bad day, especially when you can see they are trying. This could trigger a setback.

Tell them that you are proud of all the positive changes they have made in their life along the road to recovery. Your voice will be heard.

Don't talk about weight, numbers or food. This can add to the stress.

Instead, set healthy boundaries around food and mealtimes. Prepare healthy meals that are smaller portions that you can eat together.

Please know that putting too much food on the plate can be daunting and overwhelming. You can almost guarantee that your loved one is counting the calories in their mind before the plate touches the table and is already being consumed with thoughts of food and plagued with planning the purge.

Give them control and allow them to put what food they want on their plate. If they don't finish the meal, it's ok.

Don't give them a hard time. If they ate, smile at them, squeeze their hand and acknowledge that this was good.

Have an understanding that immediately after meals, the toilet is off limits for a short period. This time is one of the worst for someone living with bulimia. So, play a game or go out for a short walk together to redirect the focus.

Implement fun activities that can enhance the day. Find things to make them laugh. All these small moments of fun, laughter and love will soon grow into longer moments. This is the goal.

Bulimia is an addiction. The cyclical thoughts need to be retrained and the only way it can be done is through repetition.

Don't give up. Stay strong. I know that it seems far away right now, but recovery is obtainable.

There is a light at the end of the tunnel. Although, you may get lost in the deep depths of it. Go in and be the guide in the darkness, be the voice of encouragement, reach out your hand and support your loved one through the journey.

Remember, if there is a way into the tunnel, there must be a way out of it.

.

Made in the USA
Columbia, SC
14 September 2022

66835265R00076